THE
SHIATSU
MANUAL

THE SHIATSU MANUAL

Step-by-step techniques for a full body treatment

Gerry Thompson

Photography by Sue Atkinson

Consultant: Elaine Liechti
Director, Glasgow School of Shiatsu

 Sterling Publishing Co., Inc. New York

To Shizuko Yamomoto,
my first Shiatsu teacher.

Library of Congress Cataloging-in-Publication Data Available

2 4 6 8 10 9 7 5 3

Published 1994 by Sterling Publishing Company, Inc.
387 Park Avenue South. New York. N>Y> 10016

Originally published in Great Britain by
Headline Book Publishing, a division of Hodder Headline PLC
338 Euston Road, London NW1 3BN
under the title *The Shiatsu Manual*
Text copyright © 1994 by Gerry Thompson
Photographs copyright © 1994 by Sue Atkinson
This edition copyright © 1994 by Eddison Sadd Editions
Distributed in Canada by Sterling Publishing
c.o. Canadian Manda Group, One Atlantic Avenue, Suite 105
Toronto, Ontario, Canada M6K 3E7

AN EDDISON · SADD EDITION
Edited, designed and produced by
Eddison Sadd Editions Limited
St Chad's House
148 King's Cross Road
London WC1X 9DH

Phototypeset in Garamond ITC Light and Frutiger Roman by
Bookworm Typesetting, Manchester, England
Origination by Columbia Offset, Singapore
Printed and bound by Graficromo, S.A., Cordoba, Spain

Sterling ISBN 0–8069–0738–X

Opposite. *The oriental character* T'ai, *which means*
'great', expresses the traditional spirit of Shiatsu
and its relationship to human life.

CONTENTS

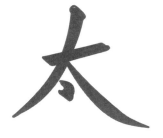

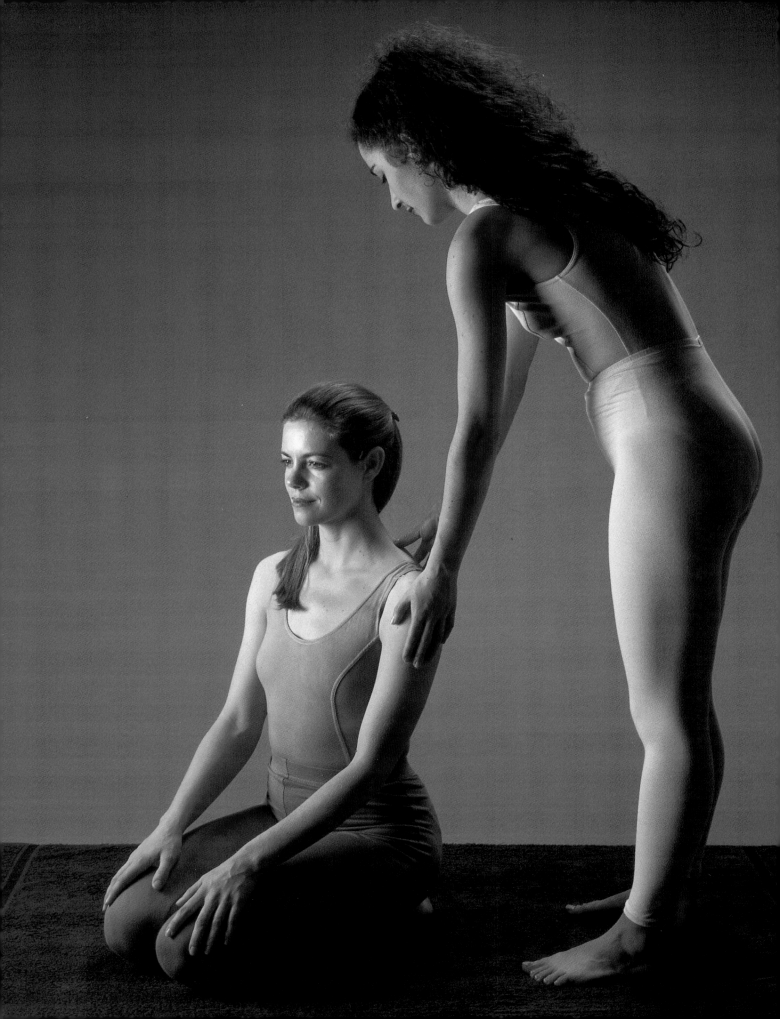

INTRODUCTION

This Introduction contains very important pointers that will help you learn the art of Shiatsu effectively; it also presents some important 'do's and don'ts' to consider when giving a Shiatsu treatment. Therefore it is strongly recommended that you read it carefully before proceeding to Part One.

Whilst building up your practical experience of Shiatsu as you work through Part One, you may wish to learn some self-treatment; various self-help routines are set out in Part Two. These can be used as exercises in their own right, or to provide a valuable warm-up before giving treatment.

Once you have practised the sequence a number of times and feel confident about giving Shiatsu treatment, move on to Part Three. There you will find a variety of additional techniques and background information that will improve your style of Shiatsu and enable you to give more versatile treatments. Incorporating these skills, you can continue to follow the Part One sequence until you no longer need to refer to the text.

If you find that Shiatsu strikes a chord with you, that you enjoy it and adapt well to it, I recommend that you attend classes. This is essential if you wish to qualify as a Shiatsu practitioner. The Resources give further information, including contact addresses, for those who wish to pursue study of Shiatsu further.

What is Shiatsu?

Shiatsu is a form of natural bodywork that uses touch to affect the body's internal vital energy flow, and so benefit health. The word 'Shiatsu' literally means 'finger pressure', but thumbs, hands and other parts of the body, such as elbows and feet, are also used. This human

Left. Giving Shiatsu treatment to the shoulders is one of the quickest ways to help your partner unwind and relax.

quality of touch is combined with an awareness of 'meridians', or channels of energy flow – the same as those used in acupuncture.

This treatment has various effects: promoting circulation and flow of lymphatic fluid, working on the nervous system, releasing deep-seated tension from the muscles and toxins from the body tissue, stimulating the hormonal system, and generally mobilizing the body's own healing abilities. Thus Shiatsu can benefit almost any ailment, including many emotional conditions. After practice at the introductory level presented in this book, treatment given to family and friends can confidently be expected to relieve tension and promote relaxation, generate energy, ease aches and pains, and help create a general feeling of well-being in body, mind and spirit.

The origins of Shiatsu

Shiatsu comes to us primarily from Japan. It is generally considered to have two main roots, both of which still fundamentally influence Shiatsu as it is practised and taught today. One source is the ancient and profound system of classical Chinese medicine, which was imported into Japan over many centuries, while the other forms a more traditional, folk-medicine approach to massage, itself a descendent of the instinctive art of healing by touch, which was handed down within families and communities in the Far East. This fusion of influences may account for the effectiveness of Shiatsu, not only as a highly sophisticated clinical therapy, but also as a simple, natural, intuitive, personal and very physical activity, well suited to a domestic situation. It is probably also why those who are relatively new to the practice of Shiatsu are able to bring benefit to those they work on, using very simple techniques they have just acquired.

Last century, Western understanding of anatomy and physiology began to gain admiration in Japan, also influencing the development of Shiatsu. Finally, the last fifteen years or so have seen a phenomenal growth in awareness and popularity for Shiatsu beyond the Orient, and particularly in Europe, the USA and Australia. Consequently, Shiatsu technique is naturally evolving in the West, in forms that are appropriate to deal with modern Western lifestyle and health issues.

How Shiatsu works

Shiatsu, in whatever form it is practised, is fundamentally a way of influencing a person's overall condition through affecting the pattern of internal energies, or 'Ki', that flow through the human body. Ki is a word that will occur often in your study of Shiatsu. It means 'vital energy', much the same as the Chinese 'chi', as in Tai Chi, or the Indian term 'prana'. When the word 'energy' is used throughout this book, it is generally in this sense and not the conventional Western usage. At first Ki may seem a rather vague concept, but it will soon become something very evident and indeed tangible to you as you practise Shiatsu. When there is something wrong with the flow of Ki in the body, then ailments manifest. Shiatsu assists in restoring the situation in three broad ways:

● removing blockages in Ki flow
● reducing excess or deficiency of Ki
● reducing relative Ki imbalances in the system.

For the time being, however, it is not essential to be able to detect these processes occurring; simple Shiatsu will still produce valuable results. Part Three looks more closely at the notion of Ki, in order to help you perceive it, so that you can make assessments about its quality and refine your technique as a result.

When Shiatsu began to be taught in the West during the late 1970s, the style of treatment that came from Japan was somewhat strong and forceful compared with the prevailing Western idea of bodywork, and this 'style' was taken to heart by many teachers and students. As a result, some people still think that receiving Shiatsu means someone walking all over your back and generally causing you a lot of pain. However, Western technique has adapted over the last decade or so,

and it is now widely accepted that good Shiatsu treatment need not be excessively painful. It is true though, that pressing certain points, where energy is imbalanced, can cause a degree of discomfort of a particular kind, which regular receivers of Shiatsu will come to recognize. It is a good idea to mention this to prospective recipients, and ask them to alert you if the treatment seems unduly painful. This leads us into the important subject of cautions to be aware of whilst giving treatment.

Cautions

There are a number of important restrictions that apply to Shiatsu, which you must be aware of *before giving any treatment*. In order to ascertain what needs to be taken into account, you will have to ask the prospective recipient some simple questions and make some accurate observations yourself, before starting the treatment. The following points can act as a mental checklist to work through before you begin:

1 Consider the recipient's basic condition and current overall state in order to determine the general tone of the treatment. This is really a matter for common sense – an elderly, frail, ill or very slimly-built person will clearly call for a lighter touch, with much less pressure all round, than someone who is sturdy, robust and in good health.

2 Discover whether the recipient has any injuries, varicose veins or partially healed surgical wounds, and avoid direct pressure on the affected areas.

3 Find out if the recipient has just eaten a heavy meal, has a fever or very high blood pressure; do not treat in these cases.

4 People with serious health problems, such as cancer, a weak heart or advanced arthritis, require treatment by a qualified practitioner.

5 In the case of female recipients, it is important to check that they do not suspect pregnancy. Do not give treatment during the first three months of pregnancy; and throughout the whole term avoid strong pressure below the knee and on certain other points mentioned in the caution boxes within the step-by-step sequence. These lie on the shoulder

near the neck, just above the inner ankle and on the hand between the thumb and forefinger (*see pages 24, 61–6 and 75*).

6 Avoid deep abdominal pressure or pelvic manipulation during menstruation.

Once you have begun the treatment:

Stop working immediately if the receiver experiences any sudden or severe pain when you press a particular point, and continue to avoid that spot throughout the treatment.

Preparing for a session

The setting: the room where you give a Shiatsu treatment should be big enough for a person to lie down and for you to walk all around them easily. There should be a 'mat' of sorts for the recipient to lie on – ideally a thin mattress or futon, though even a thick blanket will suffice: it should be wide enough for you to kneel alongside to give protection to your knees. A sheet laid on top of the futon will keep it clean. It is also useful to have some cushions or pillows handy. The room should be quiet and free from disturbances such as a ringing telephone or doorbell. Some people like to play peaceful music while giving treatment. Lighting a fire or candles, or burning incense are also very useful ways of enhancing the atmosphere. The temperature should be slightly higher than normal; although you will be moving most of the time, the receiver will tend to cool down as they fall into deep relaxation. A blanket or duvet can be spread over them for parts of the treatment. On completion, you may find that the room feels stuffy, musty or somehow slightly uncomfortable; this is due to the elimination processes that have been taking place during treatment, even if only at a level of energy discharge. You can clear the atmosphere by ventilation, by lighting a fire or by burning incense, if you had not already done so.

Yourself: the most important thing is to be inwardly calm and focused – not overtired, flustered or ill-prepared. A short preparatory relaxation or meditation session can help with this. When giving a treatment wear loose, comfortable clothing that allows you complete freedom of movement; natural fibres such as cotton are best. It is wise not to have just eaten a big meal. Make sure your hands are clean and your fingernails not too long; the thumbnails are particularly important. If you have long hair tie it up, so that it does not fall over the recipient when you are working close in.

The receiver: Shiatsu is usually received when clothed, as this facilitates contacting the underlying energy without the distraction of skin effects. The receiver's garments should also enable freedom of movement and be comfortable. Ask them to remove items such as watches, spectacles, contact lenses, jewellery, belts, shoes and any metal objects that are easily removed. They should not have just eaten a large meal, or be extremely hungry.

If this is the first session, let the receiver know a bit about what they can expect during treatment. You can say a word or two about what Shiatsu is, and mention the sequence of three positions you will be taking them through (*see page 15*). Emphasize in particular that they can become completely relaxed, and do not need to help you by moving any part of their body, apart from when you ask them to lie down or turn over. You should also advise them that some points will inevitably feel a little tender, but that they should alert you immediately if any stretch or pressure is sharply painful or distressing.

Work through the checklist on page 8 under 'cautions', to discover whether there are any health problems that will influence the treatment you are about to give, or will incur the cautions in the sequence. Some people have particular sensitivities or intolerance to touch, such as in the abdomen or toes. As you practise and learn more, you may also want to find out what the person hopes to gain from the treatment, and proceed accordingly.

It is not uncommon for recipients of Shiatsu, especially after a vigorous treatment, to experience a temporary 'reaction' in the twenty-four hours or so afterwards. This may take the form of extreme tiredness, cold-like symptoms or sometimes mild diarrhoea. The reaction is the result of toxins being released into the bloodstream before being excreted, and this can be explained to the recipient if it occurs. Sometimes a reaction can be experienced

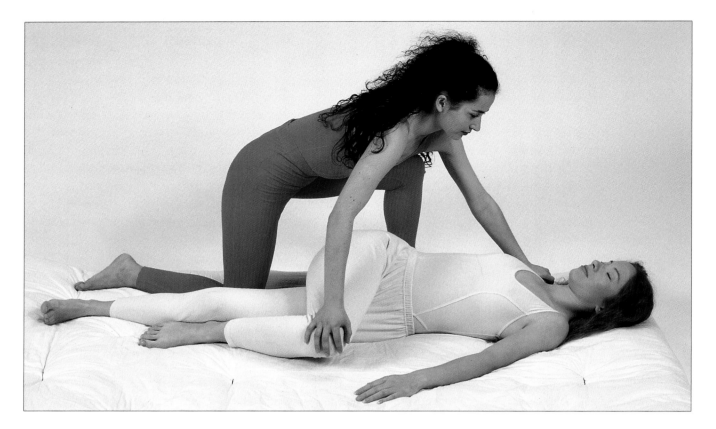

Above. *A typical overall stretch, carried out in the frequently used 'lunge' position.*
Right. *An example of pressure with the palms, given while kneeling in the 'all fours' position.*
Below. *Point work with the thumb; this produces the most intense and specific results.*

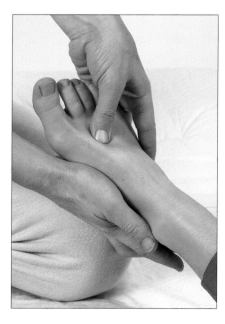

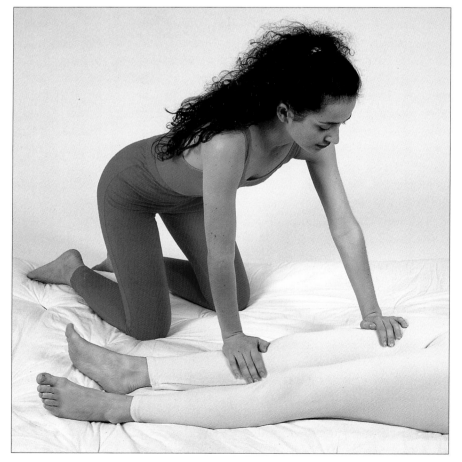

more at an emotional level, such as unaccountable temporary irritability. It is a good idea to warn the receiver about the possible reactions they may encounter.

Techniques

There is no standard procedure, or hard-and-fast routine, for a full Shiatsu treatment; rather, each practitioner and teacher has a somewhat individualized repertoire of techniques from which he or she will draw according to the requirements of each individual case. The sequence presented in Part One is a basic but comprehensive one, which incorporates commonly used elements of Shiatsu treatment. If you study Shiatsu further, this sequence will serve as a framework for other components and can be varied to suit particular circumstances. You will also naturally develop your own style as you gain experience.

Shiatsu uses pressure to affect the internal body energy or Ki, as described already, but the means used can be very diverse. The various methods include pressing, stretching, kneading, rubbing, shaking, pounding and rocking. Furthermore, there are a number of different ways that pressure can be brought to bear – with the thumbs, palms, fingers, elbows or feet. The methods in this book concentrate on thumb and palm pressure, but finger and foot pressure are also touched upon.

The most frequently used combination of these methods and tools, and the ones to become familiar with first, are:
● overall stretches
● pressure with the palms
● pressure-point work with the thumbs.
Use the upper part of the pad, rather than the actual tip. Always keep the thumb straight as you apply pressure; some people find the thumb joint is rather weak at first, but this should improve with practice.

When applying palm or thumb pressure, you will mainly be working with a method that uses the two hands in different ways – the 'working' hand leans in, moving along the required path, while the 'support' hand remains passively in one place applying moderate pressure.

All these techniques will be explained fully with step-by-step photography and detailed captions as you work your way through the treatment sequence in Part One.

How to find the points

The first thing a new Shiatsu student wonders is: 'Am I pressing the right spot?' You will, with practice, be able to tell by touch, but in the meantime the following pointers may help. The major points lie along channels or meridians, whose courses are often compared with water channels, following the natural features or 'geography' of the body. So points are usually located in 'hollows' that lie within or between bone features and muscle groups. Valuable Shiatsu treatment can be administered, however, even when you are not on a conventional 'pressure point'. The best policy is to follow the photographs in a sequence for approximate location, then work with a sense of touch for a more accurate position, but leave the study of channel and point location until you move on to Part Three.

How much pressure to use

Again, until you gain enough experience to be able to judge for yourself, there are a number of useful points to bear in mind. The best approach is to ask the recipient to let you know what he or she is feeling. Pressure should not cause severe pain, but merely a particular kind of acceptable tenderness in some sensitive places. On the other hand, if your partner is not feeling much at all then you are probably being overcautious. Generally speaking, if you follow the postural guidelines overleaf, you will be surprised at how much of your body weight can be used without causing undue discomfort. Very strong, direct pressure should not be applied to actual joints: ankles, knees, hips, elbows and shoulders.

Guiding principles in treatment

There is a certain 'style' of giving Shiatsu that produces a special quality in the treatment and the effect. In order to help you reproduce that style it has been broken down into a series of elements, which when put together characterize it. The basic components, to be

11

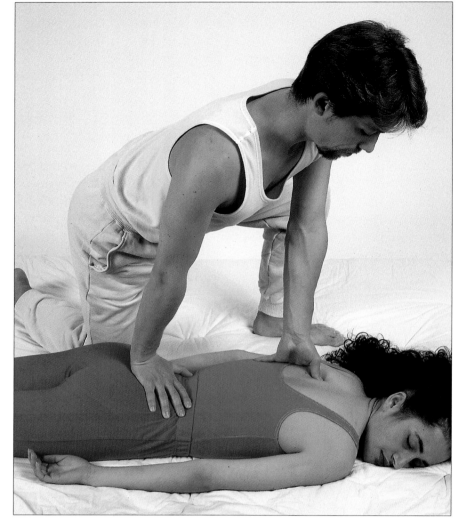

Right. *Use your body weight, not muscular effort; focus attention in your abdomen. Here, one hand is moving and working actively and the other is passive and stationary.* Below. *Keep your body in a relaxed state, and your centre of gravity low; cultivate a calm feeling.*

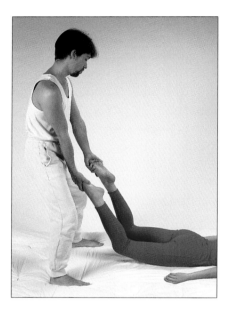

borne in mind while working, are:

1 Use your body weight, not muscular effort.
2 Keep your own body, including your arms, in a relaxed state as you work.
3 Focus attention in your abdomen, but also pay attention to your partner's response to what you are doing, for instance by watching their face. Breathing into your abdomen helps keep your own centre of gravity low, which makes you more stable and enables you to apply pressure more effectively. You can gain a physical sense of this quality by letting your belly drop and spreading your knees apart when working from a sitting position.
4 Keep the working arm straight, but not locked. For each situation you will need to position yourself far enough from the surface you are working on to do this.
5 Apply pressure by leaning into the move-

ment, as both you and your partner breathe out; and hold the position for a full out-breath.
6 Place yourself so that you can work at right angles to the surface you are treating.
7 Cultivate a calm feeling and regular rhythm.

The idea, in fact, is to achieve a sense of penetration rather than pushing. There should never be a sense of force; good Shiatsu is effortless. Generally speaking, giving Shiatsu is energizing to the giver, rather than tiring. If you incorporate all these principles, you will develop a strongly supportive technique that avoids any sensation of intrusiveness. What you are doing, really, is contacting the person's underlying Ki.

At first you may feel as though you have one hundred and one things to think about, but as time goes on and you gain experience they will all become second nature.

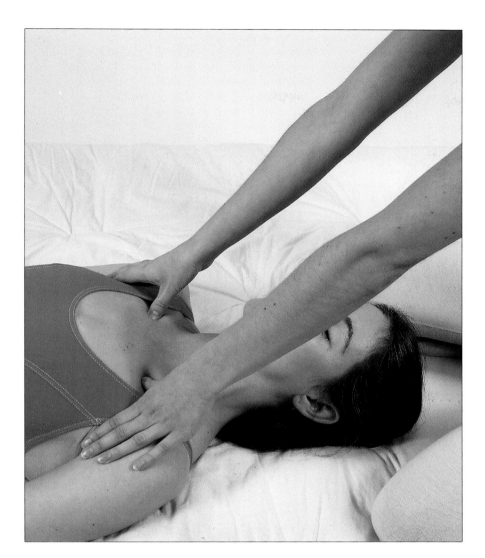

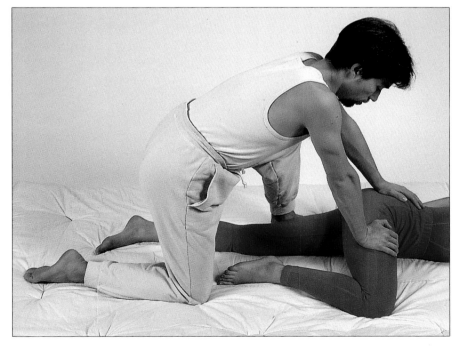

Top left. *Keep the working arm straight, though not locked.*
Bottom left. *Work at right angles to the area of the body you are treating; lean in on an out-breath and hold the position.*

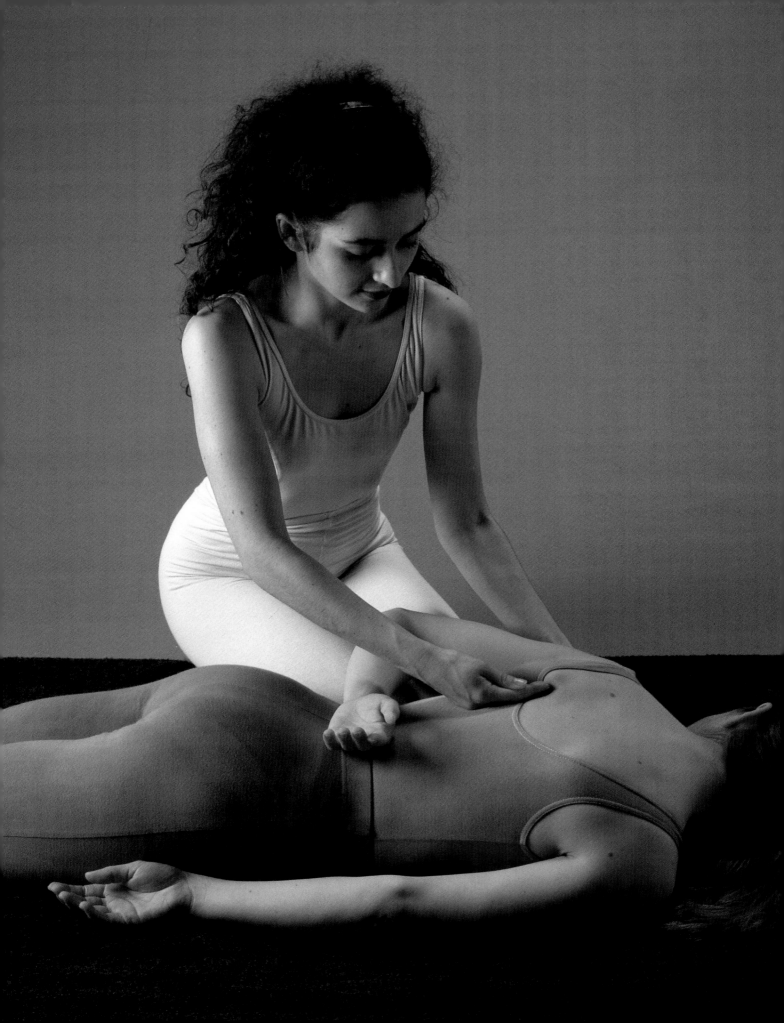

PART ONE

THE STEP-BY-STEP SEQUENCE

Before you proceed with this part, ensure that you are totally familiar with the Introduction, which includes important information to prepare you for the techniques in this section. The Shiatsu sequence is divided into ten stages, each one dealing with a different area of the body. Within the sequence there are three positions: sitting, where the shoulders are treated; face down for treatment of the whole of the back of the body; face up for work on the front of the body. The course of treatment is to work down the back of the body and up the front, following the direction of Ki flow. Each sequence tends to proceed from the general to the particular: starting with loosening movements and preparatory overall stretches, then moving on to more local palm pressure work, and finishing with pressure on specific points using thumb or fingers.

Each step is demonstrated with a photograph and detailed caption; additional photographs indicate where to apply pressure with series of points superimposed over the body. It is not essential to locate points precisely, simply follow the line indicated at approximately the intervals shown. Caution boxes indicate when you should take care with a particular technique.

Practise parts of the sequence at first, rather than trying to learn it all at once. In fact, certain sections make good shorter treatments (*see page 101*). A full body treatment should take between forty-five minutes and one hour, but it may take longer whilst you are still learning.

Left. *The back contains treatment zones for the whole body and all the major organs. Here energy is freed from the area around the shoulder-blades.*

1

THE SHOULDERS

Everyone loves having their shoulders worked on. As soon as you lay your hands on them, most people relax and sigh with delight. This is because our shoulders play such an important role in modern, urban society. They represent the ability to take responsibility, to carry a burden, to 'shoulder a load'. People who are affected by stress, and have difficulty in detaching themselves from the cause of it, whether it be work, financial difficulties or just everyday life, will almost certainly have problems in this area. Treating the shoulders brings with it the caring, sympathetic quality that is imparted when one person lays their hand on another's shoulders as a simple expression of concern or support.

In fact, the upper body is a particularly problematic zone in Western society, where there is a collective habit of concentrating energy here – constantly using the mind to solve problems. The shoulders in particular reflect an inability to focus on one issue at a time, due to a constant pressure, experienced by many people, to think about all their other problems, obligations, or things they need to do, at the same time. The shoulders are also closely associated with the neck and together they form a bridge to the head. It is the shoulders that will hold tension if there is a blockage in the flow of energy to the head.

A sedentary way of life can also cause problems; lack of movement diminishes mobility and flexibility in the shoulders. At the same time, however, excessive exercise, such as weight-training, can also create habitual tension. Treatment of the shoulders can help very directly with all these problems.

About this sequence

The shoulder treatment is carried out with the receiver in a sitting position, a more active experience for them before they lie down for the whole of the rest of the sequence and generally become more relaxed. Shoulder work begins with overall loosening-up, followed by preparatory palm pressure and tension-releasing stretches, before going on to local pressure-point work. Shoulder Shiatsu makes a convenient mini treatment on its own, as well as being a good way to begin a comprehensive session. It is an ideal means with which to introduce people to Shiatsu without them feeling at all threatened, as it can be given casually in any situation where the recipient can sit down.

Some problems that particularly benefit from this sequence include neck and shoulder tension, frozen shoulder, stiffness between shoulder-blades, upper backache, postural problems and tension headaches. Associated organs that also benefit from shoulder treatment include the intestines, gall bladder and lungs.

POINTS TO REMEMBER

- *use your body weight, not muscular effort*
- *keep your own body relaxed*
- *focus attention and breathe in your abdomen*
- *keep your working arm straight but not locked*
- *lean into each movement on the out-breath, and hold the position*
- *work at right angles to the body surface*
- *cultivate a calm feeling and regular rhythm*

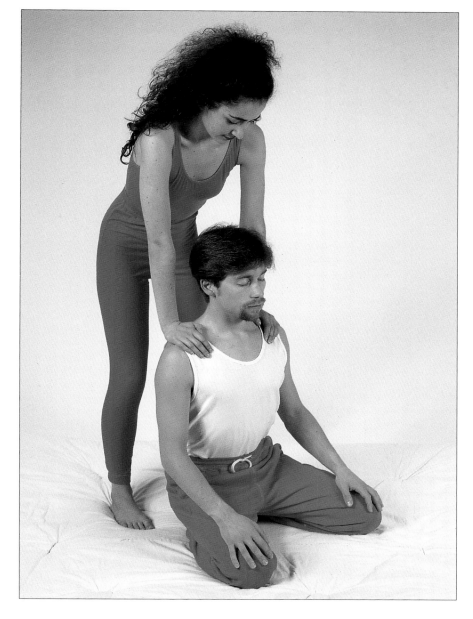

1 Ask your partner to kneel with knees spread slightly apart (*left*). If this is not comfortable due to age, stiffness or poor circulation, they can sit on the floor, with legs crossed (*bottom left*), with legs straight out (*bottom centre*) or otherwise in an upright chair without arms (*below*). This sequence proceeds with the kneeling option, so if you are using one of the alternatives you may have to adapt your working position for some of the techniques. If using a chair, for instance, you will have to adopt a standing position throughout and the stretches on pages 23–25 will not be possible. Try to keep your spine straight, especially when giving stretches; use the strength in your legs instead of bending your back. Make contact with your partner by placing your hands gently on their shoulders.

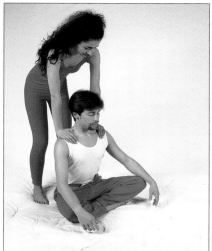

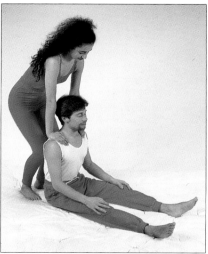

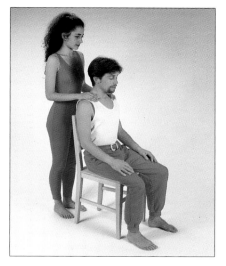

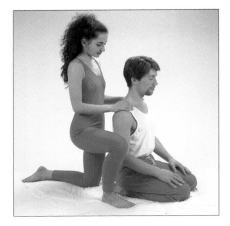

2 Kneel behind your partner with one leg raised (*right*), providing support for their back with your knee if they seem to require it. Keep both hands on your partner's shoulders for some moments, aware of making a connection between your respective energies. Your breathing should be natural and relaxed. Continue for as long as it feels appropriate.

3 Lift your partner's shoulders (*below*) and let them drop naturally with their own weight. Repeat this a couple of times, until the shoulders feel loose and heavy, and in a relaxed state. If you notice that your partner is helping you by lifting their shoulders of their own accord, point this out and try to encourage them to relax and let go.

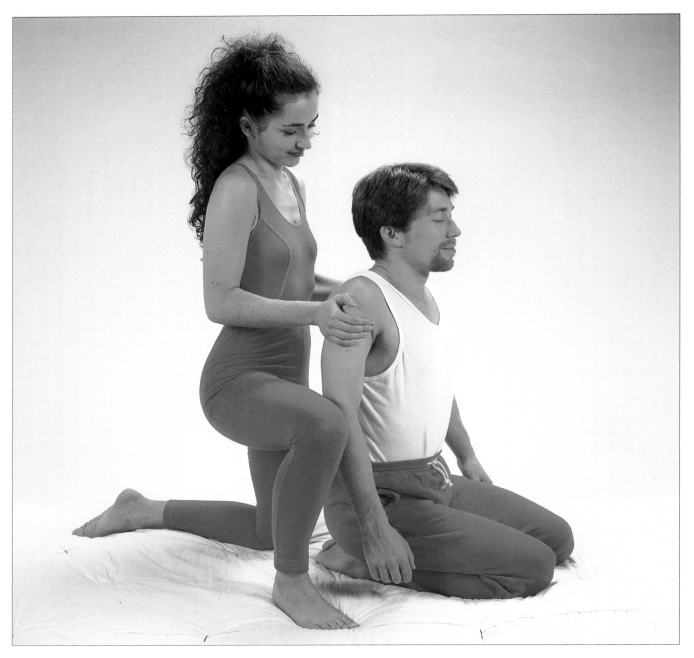

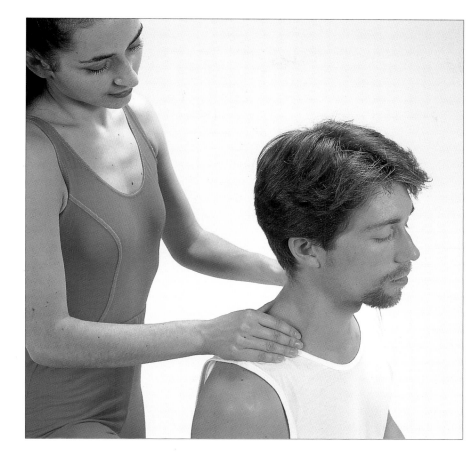

4 Begin squeezing the shoulder muscles with thumbs, fingers and palms, in a strong kneading action (*left*). As you do so, feel for the condition of the muscles – are they hard or tense? Can you detect particular spots where energy seems blocked? Do you sense good muscle tone, firm but not tight? Or perhaps there is a lack of tone, or feeling of emptiness. Make a mental note of these qualities; when you have finished the shoulder treatment check again, you will probably notice a distinct improvement.

As well as giving you information about the internal condition of the shoulders, this kneading action brings increased circulation and internal energy flow into the area, preparing it for the more concentrated techniques that follow. You can extend this action by pressing with your thumbs into the muscles on either side of the spine in the upper back.

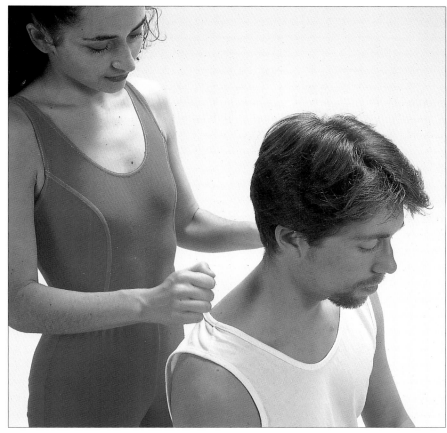

5 With loosely-held fists and keeping your wrists very floppy, pound over the shoulder muscles using the fronts of your fingers (*left*) for a minute or two. This action can be fairly vigorous as long as your partner is not feeling fragile. It helps release tension and shift blockages in Ki flow.

6 Adopt a standing position behind your partner. At this point, you can both begin to use the regular method of 'shiatsu breathing' – breathing out together as pressure is applied, taking a light in-breath as it is released, and proceeding in this relaxed rhythm.

Place your left hand on the left shoulder – this will be the fixed or 'passive' hand for the time being (*below*). Ask your partner to breathe in, and do so yourself at the same time. Then, as you both breathe out, lean down onto the right shoulder with the heel of your right hand (the 'active' hand). Lean in for the full out-breath. As you do so, keep your right arm straight, and bring your upper body weight to bear over the shoulder, rising up onto your toes if your partner is taller than you.

Repeat this four or five times at intervals, beginning near the neck and moving out along the shoulder, continuing the same pattern of breathing. Then repeat the procedure, using your left hand actively palming the left shoulder, with your right hand passively positioned on the right shoulder.

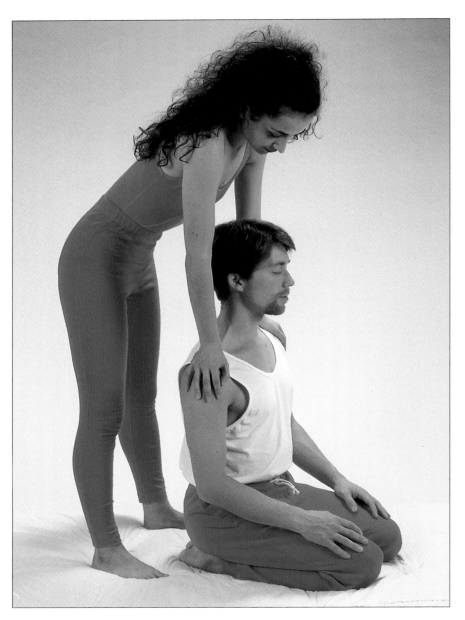

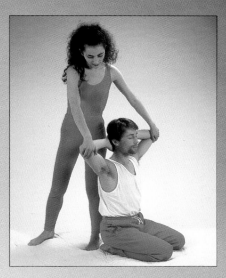

7 Still standing behind your partner, turn your body sideways so that your thigh or hip is placed centrally against your partner's spine (*above*). Position your feet far enough apart to give you a stable base and ask your partner to place their hands behind their neck, with the fingers interlocked, and simply to relax their arms. Place your hands one in front of each of their elbows.

Breathe in, and on the out-breath smoothly pull back on the elbows to a comfortable stretch (*left*). This is helpful in releasing tension, especially between the shoulder-blades and in the shoulder joints.

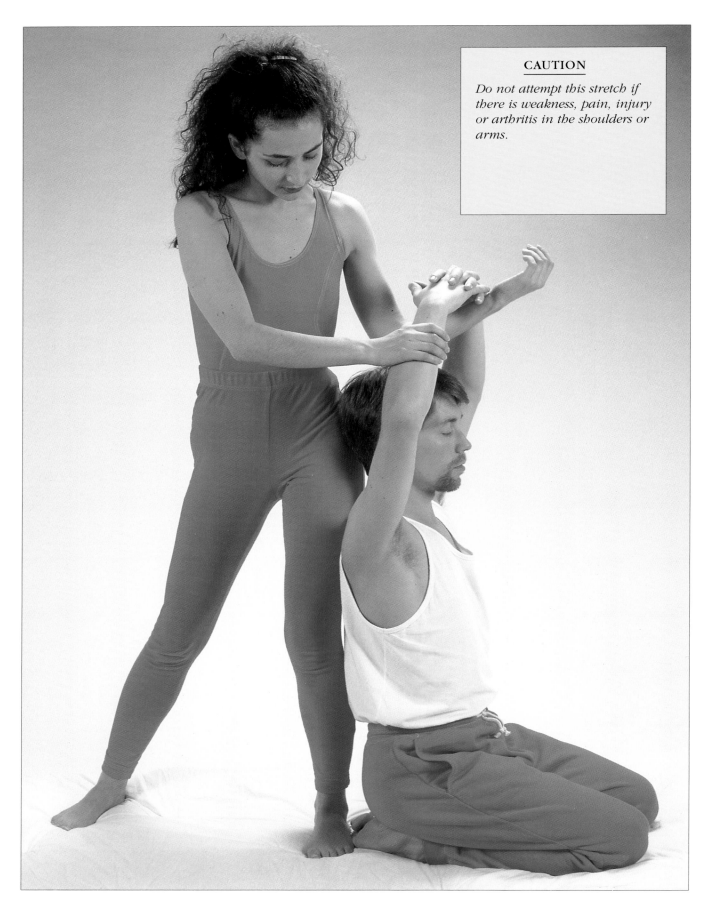

8 Stand behind your partner as before, with your thigh or hip meeting their spine. The key to this stretch is to keep this point of contact central throughout, stopping your partner twisting around. Keep your feet widely spaced to give you a firm base.

Ask your partner to interlink their fingers and raise their arms overhead. Pass your arm through the loop (*opposite page*). Rest their hands on your shoulder (*right*). Keeping in contact with their body, tilt gently away, pivoting at the

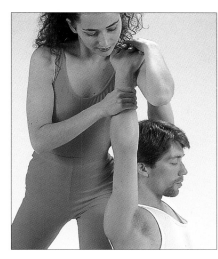

hip, so that their arms straighten. If you need to lower your body in relation to theirs, place your outside leg further away still.

Explain to your partner that this stretch will lift their body slightly, and that they should allow their arms to straighten and their weight to fall, so that their hips will come off their legs. Ask them to breathe in and do so yourself at the same time. Now pivot your body further (*below*), making sure that your legs are doing the work. Hold the stretch for the full out-breath.

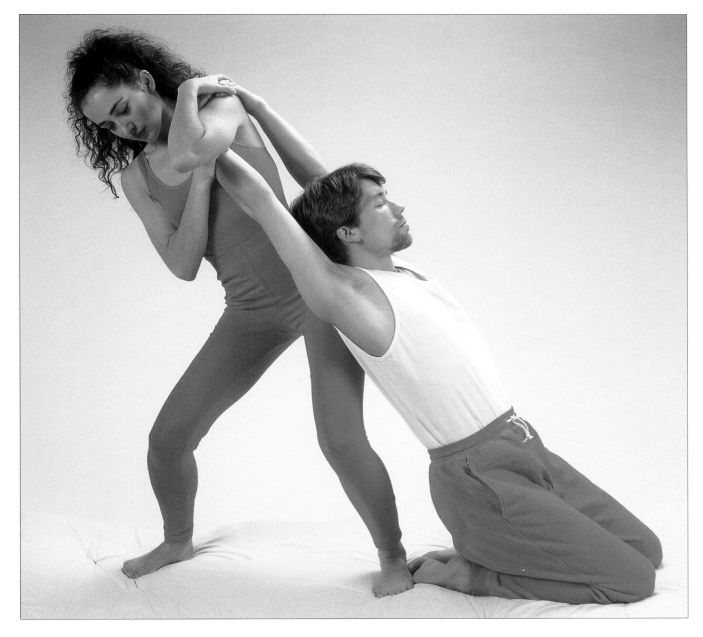

9 Position yourself at right angles to your partner's left side, with your left hand resting on the front of the shoulder (*below*). Using your right thumb, press firmly into the shoulder muscle beginning near the neck (*far right*). Make sure you keep your right arm straight as you do this, by adjusting your distance from your partner accordingly. Repeat at intervals on the pressure points along the top of the shoulder muscles (*top left, opposite page*). Then move to your partner's right side and repeat.

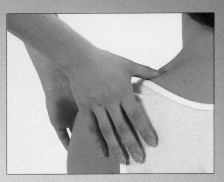

CAUTION

Avoid these points during pregnancy as they can induce labour.

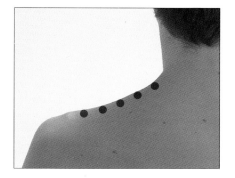

Shoulder pressure points
The points worked on in step 9 run along the top of the shoulder muscles, from the neck to the outside of the shoulder (*left*). Press at intervals of a thumb's width. Pay special attention to places where you feel a blockage.
Benefits: releases tension in shoulders and neck; relieves related headaches; also aids the gall bladder.

10 Knead the shoulder muscles again to assess the difference your treatment has made. Then with your fingers, brush several times along the shoulders and on to the back (*below*), sweeping outwards from the neck. This 'smooths out' patterns of energy in the areas you have been working on, where there may have been energy blockages and imbalances.

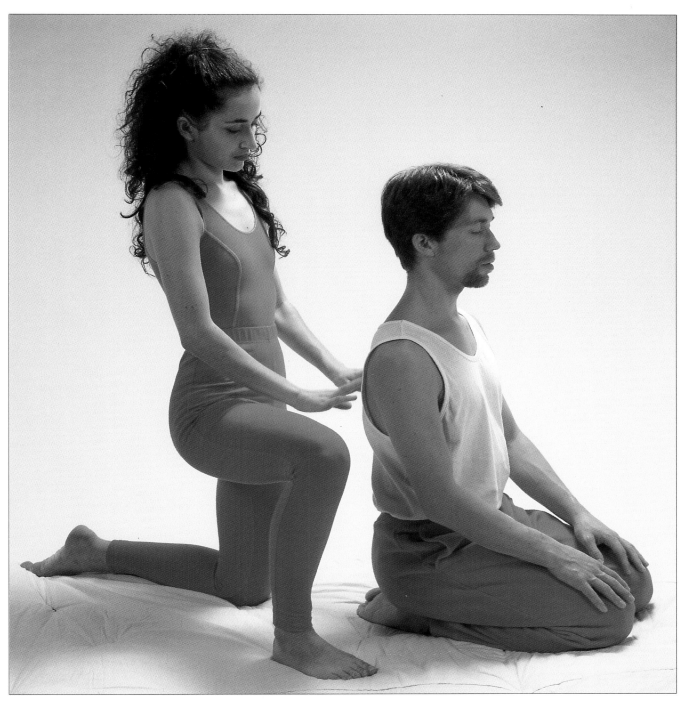

2

THE BACK

The back is in many ways the most significant part of the body to treat with Shiatsu. This lesson introduces the basic Shiatsu techniques that will be applied throughout the rest of the sequence. You will find it particularly good for practising the guiding principles for treatment (*see pages 11–13*).

Treating the back brings benefit to the whole of the body; it is a 'mirror' of the total system, with a series of zones and pressure points that have precise correspondences to each of the major organ systems. Broadly speaking, each zone of the spine corresponds to the organs that are placed at the same level in the abdominal cavity. This means that spinal problems themselves are bound up with the health of the corresponding organs; if specific back problems are not to recur, it is important that these underlying causes are discovered and treated, and that internal Ki energies are corrected. General treatment of the back will help correct these Ki imbalances.

Therefore the back is a classic example of how each part of the body both reflects and affects other parts and other functions. So, as with the shoulders, working on the back will eventually tell you a lot about the condition of the whole system as well as providing the treatment to help improve its functioning.

The back is a robust structural unit consisting of the spine and ribs, providing support to the upper body and protecting the vital organs. It often holds great tension; this can be due to overwork or other stress, lack of exercise, postural habit, protection of weak areas, or a kind of 'armouring', which is often associated with personal matters from the past.

Most people feel at ease about being touched on the back, so you can lean in with your whole weight – apart from where there is known injury or local weakness – and this will help release these tensions.

A healthy back is supple with good muscle tone; the spine should not project or recede excessively and the muscle should appear symmetrical (both visually and by touch) on either side of the spine.

About this sequence
The sequence here commences work with the recipient lying face down. We start with preliminary loosening techniques over the back of the body, including the large muscles of the buttocks – the Gluteus Maximus – and the backs of the legs. These promote relaxation, and are followed by some stretches for release of more local tension. You then follow the classic Shiatsu procedure of palm work and pressure-point work with the thumbs, working from the top of the spine down to the buttocks.

POINTS TO REMEMBER

- *use your body weight, not muscular effort*
- *keep your own body relaxed*
- *focus attention and breathe in your abdomen*
- *keep your working arm straight but not locked*
- *lean into each movement on the out-breath, and hold the position*
- *work at right angles to the body surface*
- *cultivate a calm feeling and regular rhythm*

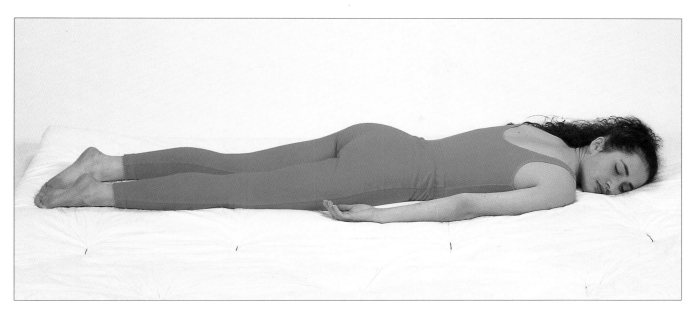

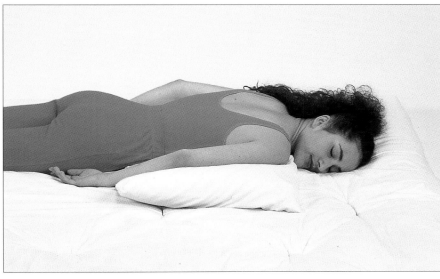

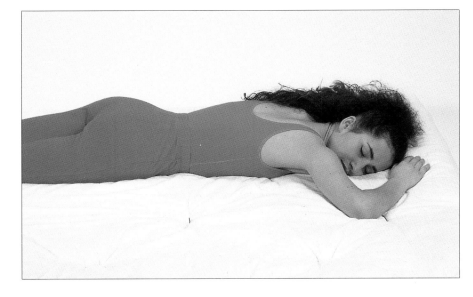

1 Ask your partner to lie face
down. Make sure that their
position enables you to kneel all
the way around them, including
above the head and below the feet.
The traditional position for Shiatsu
is with the arms down by the sides
and the head turned to one side
(*above*); alternatively, if the
receiver's neck is stiff or the back
is tense, a supporting cushion or
pillow can be of great benefit
(*left*). This should be placed under
the chest and below the chin, not
under the face, which would
increase rather than lessen pressure
on the neck, and would close
rather than open the upper back.
If the ankles are very stiff, another
cushion can be placed under them.
Many people prefer to receive
Shiatsu with the arms positioned
above the head (*left*), especially if
the neck is stiff; this is all right too.

CAUTION

*This position is unsuitable
during advanced pregnancy.*

27

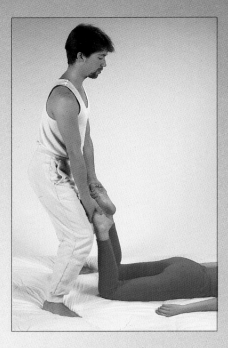

2 Keeping your own back straight, lift your partner's feet (*above*) and take the weight of their lower body. Lift until the pelvis is raised off the mattress, then swing the lower body from side to side three or four times (*left*), or more if the body seems tense. If you notice that the knee joints are locked, remind your partner to keep relaxing and 'letting go'. Finish by drawing the feet away from the head horizontally as you replace the lower body on the mattress.

3 Standing astride your partner, pick up the hands and draw the arms towards you (*below*), replacing them on the mattress. This ensures that the shoulders are in an open position and not hunched up close to the neck.

Remind your partner that they should become completely relaxed during the sequence that is to follow, and that you do not want them to 'help' you by moving any part of their body voluntarily. Do let them know, however, that they may turn their head from time to time, to avoid stiffness. It is a good idea to remind your partner to let you know if they experience any excessive or sharp pain during the treatment.

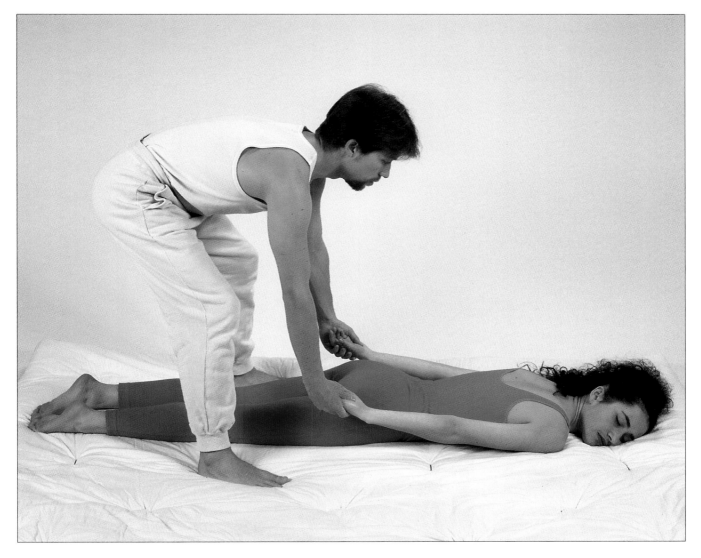

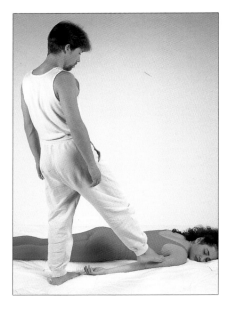

4 Move to one side of your partner, positioning yourself close enough to reach them with your foot. Begin pressing and wobbling along the upper arm with the ball of your foot (*above*). To do this, press briefly, then vibrate your foot making the flesh quiver. This loosens tension and promotes Ki flow in a preparatory way. It also provides an opportunity to feel energy blockages and muscle tension. Work from the top of the arm to the palm, but do not put firm pressure on the shoulder, elbow or wrist. Treat each area two or three times.

5 Repeat this procedure with the buttock (*right*), pressing into the muscle and around the pelvic bone. You can use a stronger action here. Look out for tension, and make a mental note of it for local pressure-point work later. Tension in this area is very common, and can often be associated with sexual issues. Work over this area two or three times.

CAUTION

Proceed gently if your partner is old or frail. Do not press directly on joints, local injuries or varicose veins.

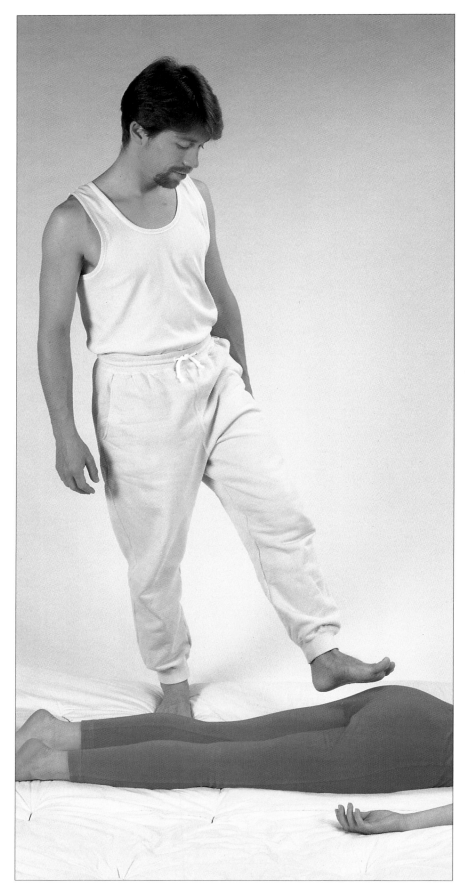

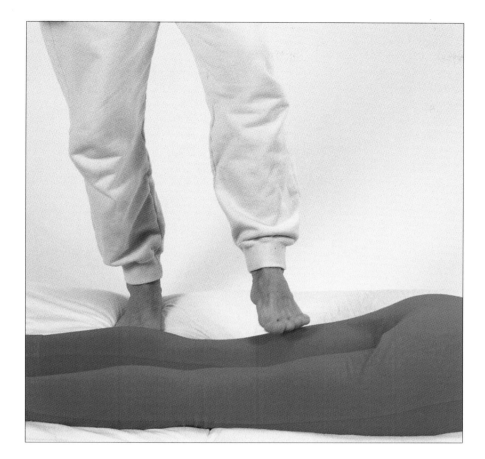

6 Continue pressing and wobbling on to the back of the thigh (*left*). Skip over the knee and proceed to the calf (*bottom left*), which is another very common area of muscular tension and 'armouring'. You can spend a little longer on areas like this. Then carry out steps 4–6 on the other side of the body, starting with the arm and working down to the calf.

Use the ball of the foot throughout this process. If you have trouble with balance, it will help to place your back foot further away from your partner, thus widening your base by spacing your legs further apart. Focusing attention in your abdomen will also help with balance.

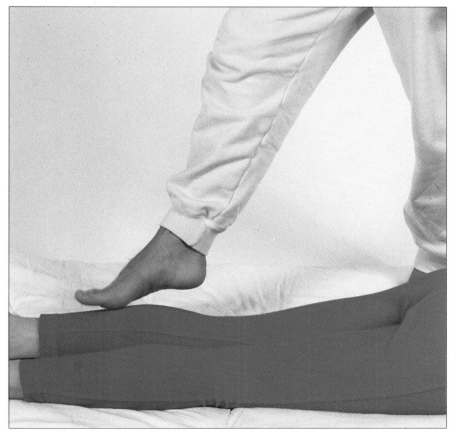

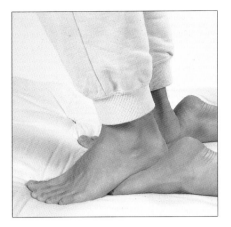

7 Now stand at your partner's feet, facing away from them, place your feet, one at a time, across theirs (*left*). Now shift your weight from side to side, pressing your heels into their soles. This opens up and releases tension in the feet. Make sure, however, that you do not put too much pressure on the ankles, especially if there is a gap under them. To avoid this, if you are not working on a soft surface, provide a cushion under the ankles.

8 Standing parallel to your partner's hips, place the ball of your foot on the sacrum. Rock the pelvis from side to side by simply pushing away, waiting for it to rock back, and immediately pushing away again (*below*). In this way you will find that person's natural rhythm, which you will recognize by the minimal effort required. This exercise promotes relaxation by sedating the nervous system. You only need to do this from one side of the body.

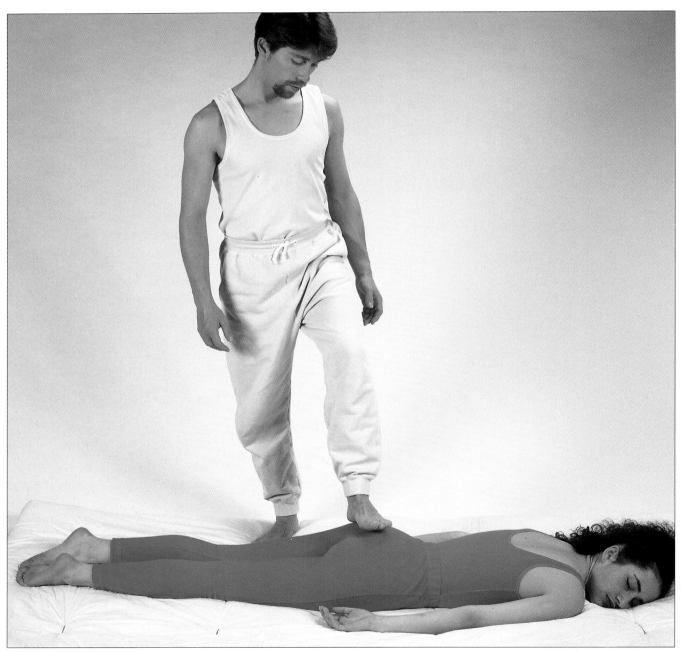

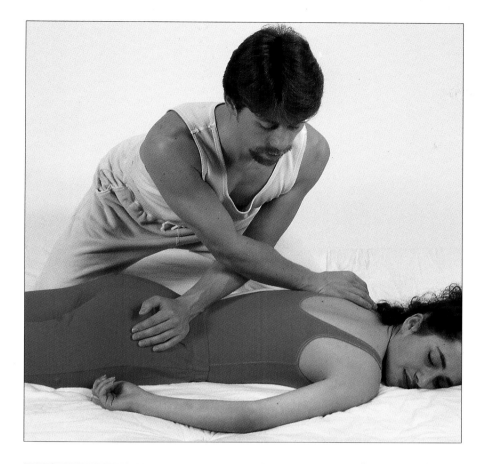

9 Kneel opposite the middle of your partner's back, with your knees spread to lower your centre of gravity. Crossing your arms, place your right hand against the bottom edge of your partner's left shoulder-blade, cupping it with the heel of your palm to gain purchase against it. At the same time, place the heel of your left hand against the top of your partner's right hip-bone (*left*). Now, lean forward on an out-breath and bring your body weight down and over your partner, which will push your hands apart and produce a strong diagonal stretch between the two points of contact. Repeat this twice more. Then shift your right hand to the right shoulder-blade, and your left hand to the left hip-bone, and stretch three times.

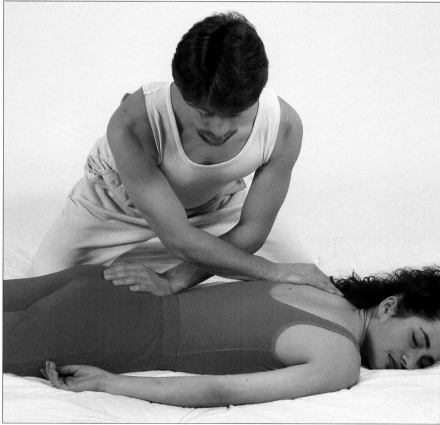

With your arms still crossed, this time place your right hand on the left shoulder-blade and your left hand on the left hip-bone (*left*). Lean in three times as before, this time producing a lateral stretch. Then reach further over and work with the right shoulder and hip, completing the four-fold series of stretches.

The effect of these stretches should come from your whole body weight and not from muscular effort in your shoulders or arms. The stretches are very helpful in opening up the back and releasing tension, prior to the more specific work which is about to begin.

10 Check over the length of the back, down each side of the spine, in the hollow that runs between it and the lateral muscles; use either your fingertips (*right*) or your thumb (*bottom right*). Look for areas or points that feel tight or blocked, different on one side to the other, or just seem to stand out no matter how ill-defined that may seem to you at present. Also practise quickly running your hands down both sides of the spine, and just see where your hand stops because you feel something 'different'. Make a mental note of any such features to pay special attention to with palm and point work. Making a habit of checking in this way will help you develop sensitivity to Ki patterns.

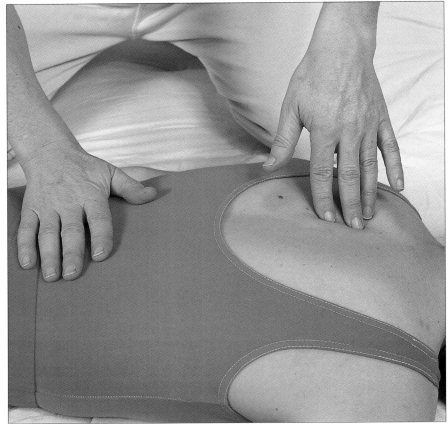

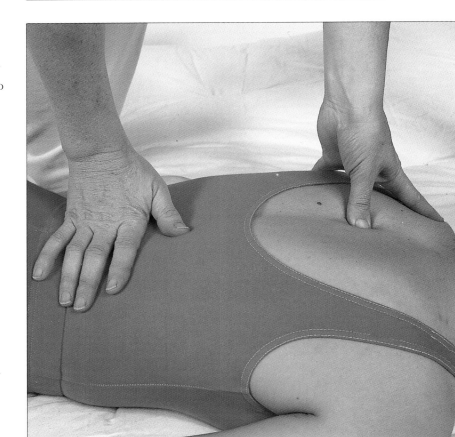

11 Remaining on the same side, come up on to one knee alongside your partner's back. Make sure that their head is turned away from you. Place your partner's nearside hand in the small of their back. Then place one hand under your partner's shoulder and lift up; as you do so, you will notice that this raises and loosens the shoulder-blade, making it more prominent and distinguishing it from the rest of the back (*right*). Starting at the lower edge of the blade, begin to press in underneath it. Use your hand with the palm up

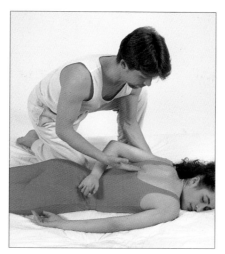

and the fingers held rigidly, rather like the blade of a knife (*bottom left*); press in on the out-breath as usual. Move around the edge of the blade towards the top; you will usually find that the area at the top feels tighter and less open than the bottom, so concentrate on this area. You can follow this by turning your hand over and using your thumb to work around the area following the same line of points shown in the photograph below. This is particularly useful if the area is very tight. Go to the other side of the back and repeat.

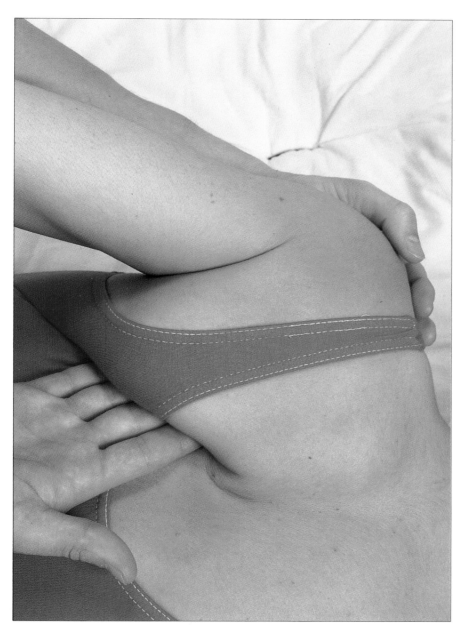

Shoulder-blade pressure points
The points used in step 11 run around the outer edge of the shoulder-blade (*above*). Press at intervals of a thumb's width. *Benefits: helps to release tension surrounding the shoulder-blades. Pressure on these points also assists the bladder.*

35

12 Shift to a kneeling position opposite the middle of your partner's back, far enough away to be able to lean in with your body weight (*right*). Place one palm on the sacrum, the flat, triangular bone below the waist; this hand will remain stationary. With your other hand, lean into the upper back on the out-breath, keeping your palm flat on the back and the heel of your hand pressing into the channel next to the spine on your side. Move down the spine in this way. When you are about half-way down, switch to palming with the other arm, keeping the previously working arm passive. Repeat this twice more. Then move to your partner's other side and repeat there.

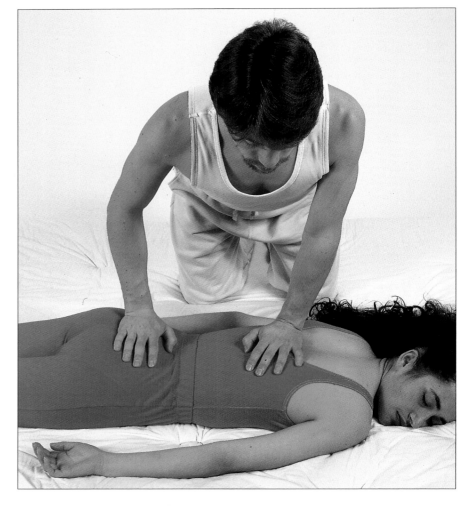

Back palming points

Approximate palming positions are shown here (*right*). Work from the upper back, right down on to the sacrum, at intervals of about one palm width to cover the whole area. Do not put pressure on the neck. Pay special attention to areas you noticed while checking in step 10, especially if there was a definite feeling of tension or blockage, and give extra treatment to these spots.
Benefits: helpful for back-ache and minor back problems, often providing a degree of helpful readjustment. Palming the back also benefits all the major organs in general, and the bladder in particular.

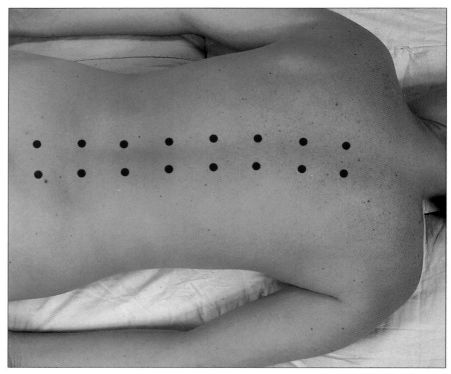

13 Move to a kneeling position above your partner's head. You will now begin to go over the areas just treated, this time with thumb pressure. Remember to use the upper part of the pad, rather than the tip, and to keep the thumbs straight. Follow the same channels between the spine and the muscles, this time treating both sides at once. Lean in with your full body weight unless the cautions opposite apply. Go down the back as far as is comfortable from your present position, before switching positions to continue in step 14. The approximate line of points is shown on page 39.

14 Move around so that you are kneeling alongside your partner's waist, in the frequently used 'lunge' position. Here you can continue where you left off with step 13, proceeding down the spine on to the sacrum. Follow the lines of points shown opposite, treating the channels on both sides of the spine from the same position on one side of the body.

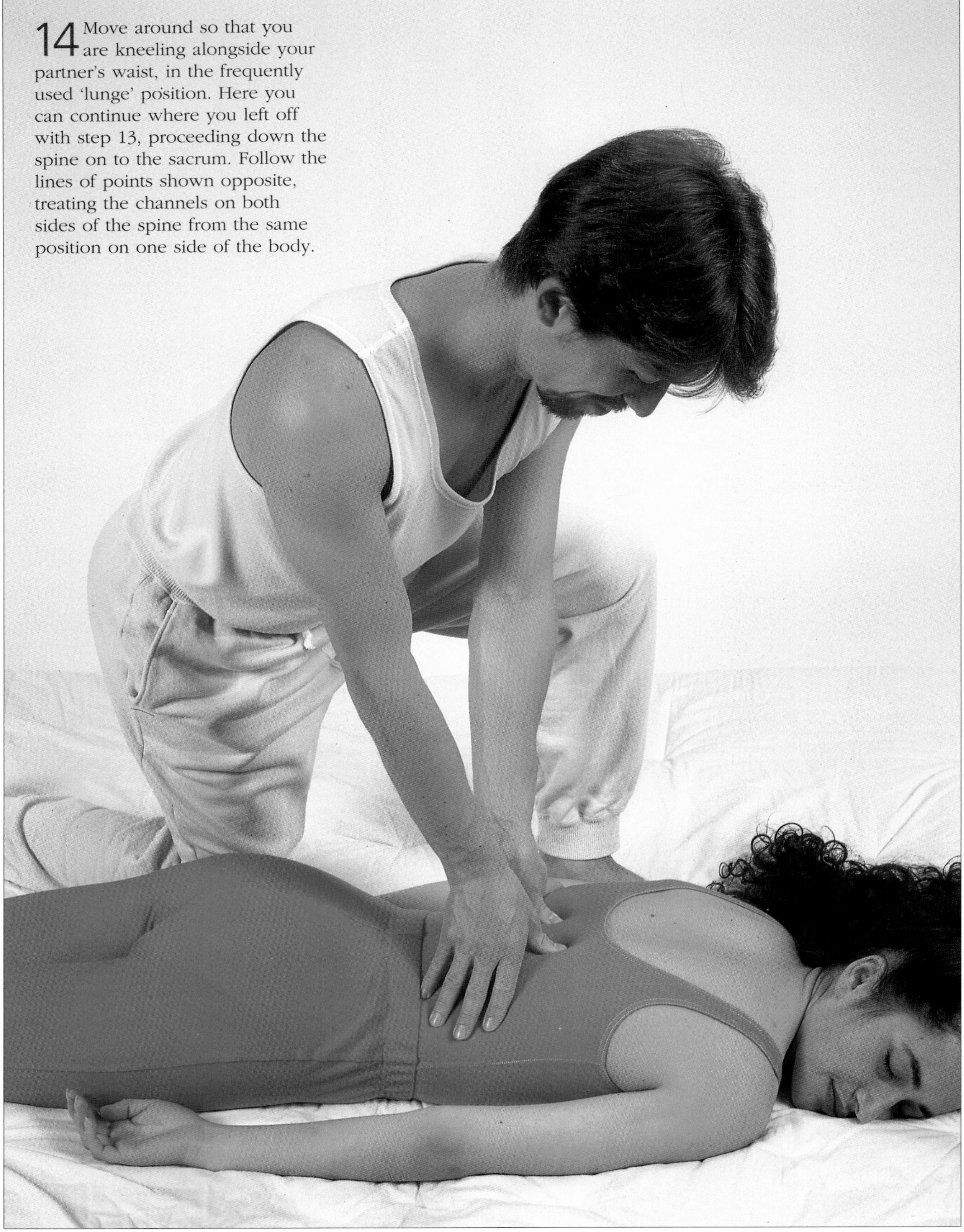

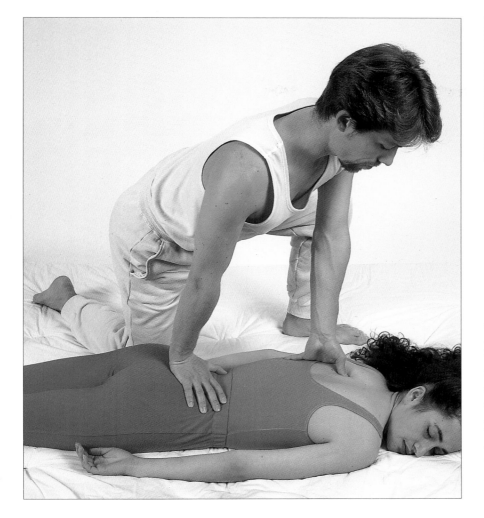

CAUTION

Never lean on the spine itself. Use light pressure if your partner is weak, elderly or has a back injury.

15 Staying in the same position, go over the same area again, this time with one line of thumb pressure points at a time. Use whichever arm is most comfortable for you as the active or working arm, positioning yourself accordingly, keeping the other stationary on the sacrum (*left*). As before, move downwards from the upper back, along the lines shown below. Again, you can treat both channels from the same position on one side of the body.

Back pressure points
The pressure points used in steps 13, 14 and 15 are shown here. Work at intervals of approximately one thumb width, from the upper back down on to the sacrum (*left*). You will find that the 'channel' peters out as you reach the sacrum. Instead you will find small hollows here on the flat, triangular bone. Go over tense or blocked areas several extra times, and lean in more strongly if blockages do not seem to respond to lighter pressure.
Benefits: helpful for back-ache and minor back problems, again providing a degree of helpful readjustment, plus more accurate treatment of aches and pains in the back. Pressure-point work on the back also benefits all the major organs and the bladder in particular.

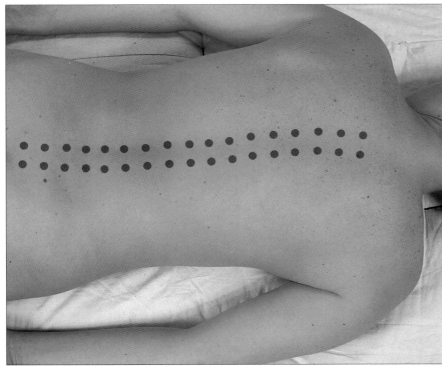

3

THE BACKS OF THE LEGS

The lower half of the body brings in some distinctive issues, both physical and emotional, that affect Shiatsu treatment. The oriental understanding of health relies on an awareness of a series of internal energy centres or 'chakras', each with a different significance. The legs connect to the sacral chakra, which is connected with issues of being 'grounded', or rooted in reality, with self-esteem, sexual and physical vitality, and with the ability to absorb life's shocks without being completely thrown off-balance. The legs can also literally carry us forward or help us run away. From a metaphysical point of view then, problems in the legs are involved with issues of 'moving forward' or 'making progress' in life, or with the ability to escape from things.

Treating the legs can have an effect on all these aspects, as well as on more physical matters. Treating the lower body generally brings the receiver more 'into the body', which is often beneficial in a society which is overly centred in the head or mind. Furthermore, traditional oriental doctors believe that deterioration of overall health with ageing begins in the legs, as they are used less and Ki flow through them decreases. Having a sedentary job and driving everywhere, instead of walking and taking regular exercise, will clearly bring on this deterioration earlier.

The buttocks too can be adversely affected by an inactive lifestyle, resulting in the stagnation of Ki. They are also often affected by tension from clenching. This can be connected with anger, aggression or sexual anxiety. Half of the classical Chinese energy channels, or meridians, begin or end in the legs (*see pages 128–30*). Therefore the legs have a particular relevance to the corresponding organs. In this sequence, the legs are worked on in two parts, separated by treatment of the feet. The backs of the legs are treated first, then the feet, then the fronts of the legs. As already mentioned, the back of the body can express a person's relationship to their past, and this can sometimes appear in the backs of the legs as extreme tension or 'armouring'.

About this sequence
The sequence for the backs of the legs begins with palming and goes on to more specific thumb pressure-point work, thus continuing the previous sequence down the back of the body, by treating in turn the buttocks, thighs and calves. This relates particularly to the bladder. A new position is then adopted to enable a similar sequence of treatment to the outside of the leg, which governs the gall bladder. These two procedures are applied, in turn, to one leg and then the other.

POINTS TO REMEMBER

- *use your body weight, not muscular effort*
- *keep your own body relaxed*
- *focus attention and breathe in your abdomen*
- *keep your working arm straight but not locked*
- *lean into each movement on the out-breath, and hold the position*
- *work at right angles to the body surface*
- *cultivate a calm feeling and regular rhythm*

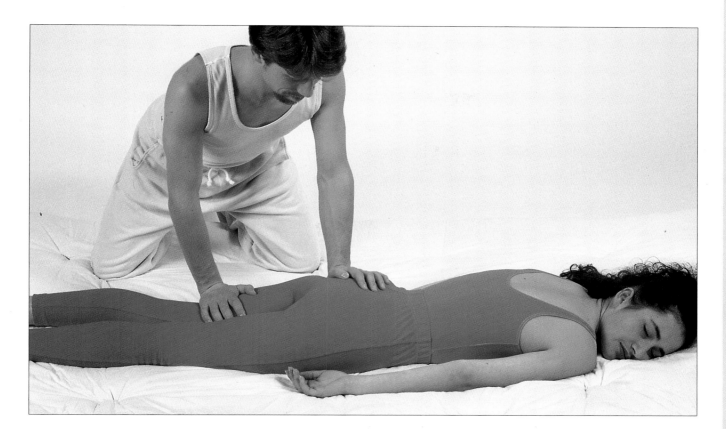

1 Kneel beside your partner's knee (*above*); from here you will be able to treat the whole leg. Lean in with your whole body weight from the side, with your palm over the buttock, keeping the other hand passive on the thigh. Work over the whole area of the buttock, especially concentrating on the lower rim of the pelvis, treating all lines of points three times.

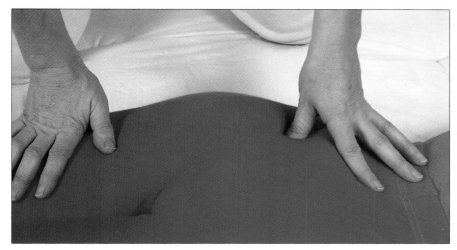

2 Cover the same area with thumb pressure (*above*). Again work around the rim of the pelvis with direct pressure in under the bone. You can work strongly in this area, unless there is a local problem, such as sciatica. The four lines of points to work on are indicated on the right. As usual, pay particular attention to blocked or stagnated points. Remain on the same side to continue work down the back of the leg.

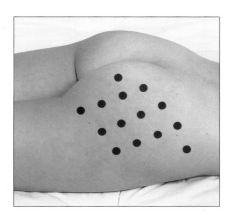

Buttock pressure points
Thumb pressure points for the buttocks are shown here (*left*). The points around the pelvis will feel tender on many people, but are valuable release points. You can lean even more strongly into the other points on the Gluteus Maximus muscle. Press at intervals of a thumb's width.
Benefits: helps hip problems, bladder and gall bladder problems, and helps alleviate sexual tension.

41

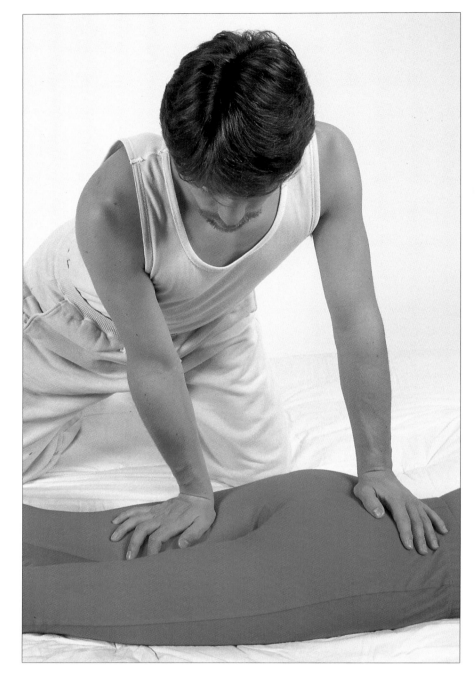

3 The previously working hand now becomes passive, remaining on the sacrum. Palm down the centre of the back of the thigh with your other hand (*right*), at intervals of a palm width, to cover the whole area as far as the knee, but without putting pressure on the knee joint. Lean in from directly above the area you are treating, again using your whole body weight.

4 Thumb down the back of the thigh (*right*), again along the centre line, and leaning in from directly above with your body weight. The line of points to follow is shown at the bottom of the opposite page. As usual, pay particular attention and give extra treatment to points that seem blocked or stagnated.

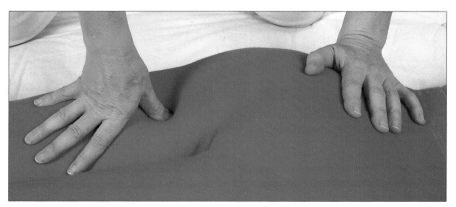

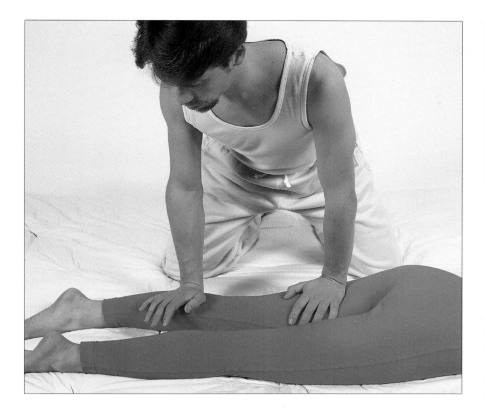

CAUTION

Avoid applying your full weight to the knees or ankles and avoid pressure on varicose veins. Do not work below the knee in early pregnancy.

5 Move the passive hand to the back of the thigh, and palm down the centre of the back of the calf (*left*) as far as the ankles, at intervals of a palm width, leaning your body weight directly from above. Do not apply direct pressure on the ankle.

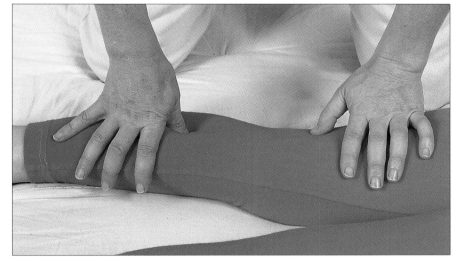

6 Go over the same area with thumb pressure (*left*). Again follow the central line indicated bottom left, as far as the ankle.

Then, when you have completed the treatment for one leg, move to the other side of your partner, kneel beside the knees and repeat steps 1–6.

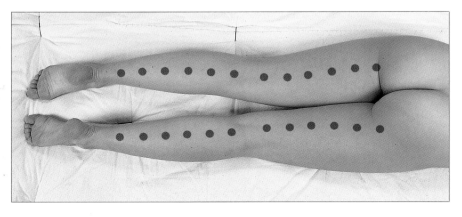

Backs of legs pressure points
Press the pressure points (*left*) at intervals of one thumb width, avoiding the knee joints and ankles. Points about half-way down the calf are sometimes particularly tender, so adjust the pressure if it is too strong. Repeat each line of pressure three times.
Benefits: helpful for aching, stiffness or joint pains in the legs and hips. Also particularly assists functioning of the bladder.

43

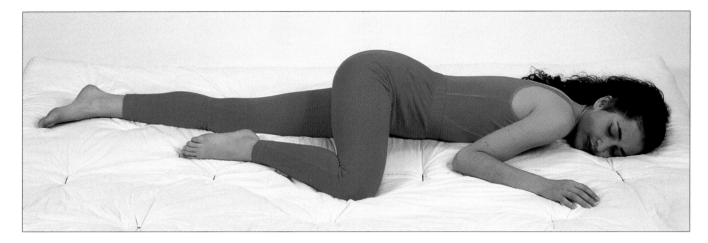

7 Ask your partner to assume the 'recovery position' (*above*), by turning the head to one side and spreading the arm out alongside, and at the same time tilting the pelvis back and drawing the knee up level with the hip. The other arm can be down by the side. This is the position for receiving treatment on the outside of the legs, beneficial to the gall bladder.

8 Adopt the lunge position, with your forward foot on the far side of your partner's body, and palm down the centre of the outer thigh (*right*). Keep your passive hand on your partner's hip.

9 Thumb along the same line (*below*), which would roughly correspond to the outer seam of a garment (*see opposite page*).

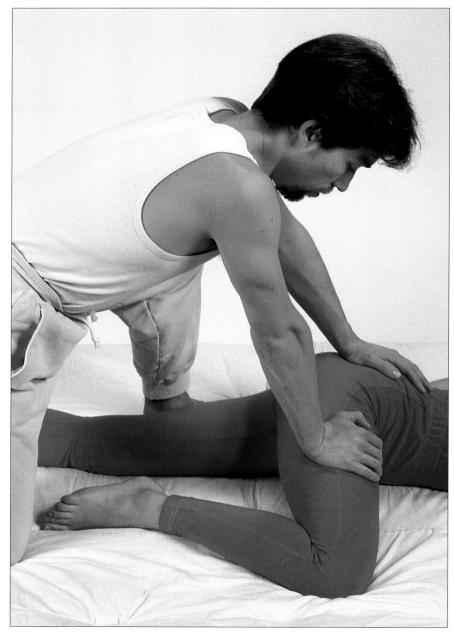

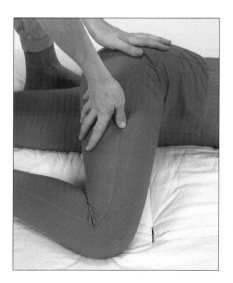

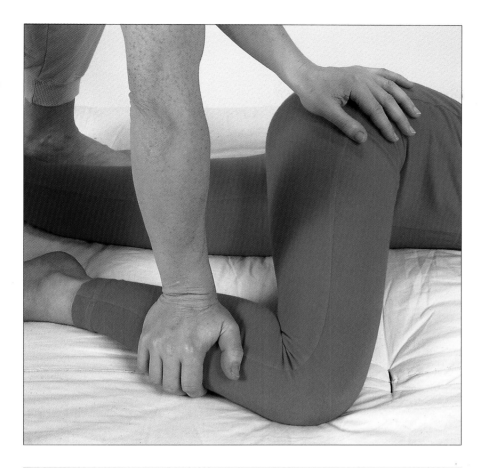

10 Remaining in the same position, palm down the centre line of the outside of the lower leg (*left*), at intervals of a palm width. Again lean in and apply pressure perpendicular to the surface. Work down to the ankle.

11 Thumb down the same line (*below*), following the points shown bottom left.
Then ask your partner to straighten that leg and roll over on to the other side, raise the other leg and repeat steps 8–11.

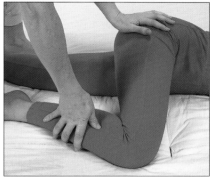

CAUTION

Avoid applying pressure where there are varicose veins. Do not work below the knee during early pregnancy.

Outer leg pressure points
The points for treatment of the outer leg are shown (*left*). Proceed, as usual, at intervals of about a thumb width to cover the whole line, and give extra treatment to areas that you feel require it. The points on the outer thigh are sometimes extremely tender; if so, work more lightly but repeat the procedure a couple of extra times.
Benefits: particularly assists functioning of the gall bladder.

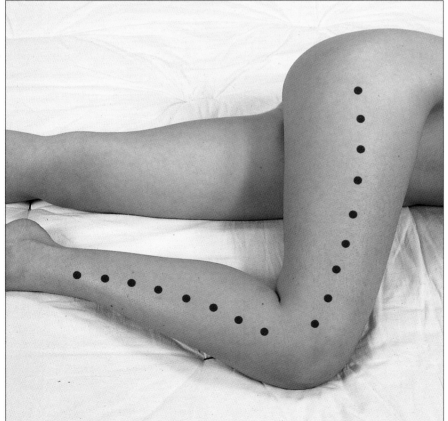

4

THE FEET

The feet are, literally and figuratively, our foundation, and relate to corresponding fundamental life issues; the condition of the feet often reflects the state of basic life matters for each individual. They also reflect the condition of the whole body, so you can get a good idea of how a person is by examining their feet. In fact, the feet can be used to treat the whole body, which has become an art in itself – reflexology. Healthy feet are strong but supple, with straight but flexible toes and well-curved arches. Treatment of the feet also draws energy away from the upper body and head, helping to ground the individual.

There are many nerve-endings in the feet, and most people find the treatment a pleasurable experience, especially since the feet are relatively passive, used to being put under pressure, often restricted in shoes, and generally taken for granted. Some people have highly sensitive feet so watch out for signs of nervousness or discomfort as you work. The foot sequence on its own makes an excellent mini treatment.

About this sequence
The feet can be treated with or without socks, although initially it may be easier to find your way around bare feet. The sequence follows on from work on the backs of the legs, and naturally falls into two sections, separated by the receiver turning over, and runs into the treatment of the front of the body. Work starts in each case with overall loosening, moving on to point work and then detailed treatment of the toes. Apart from local problems, such as tired or aching feet, fallen arches, foot or ankle injuries, tendonitis, callouses, corns and bunions, treating the feet particularly helps with problems in the head and neck.

1 Sit or kneel below your partner's feet, close enough so that you can pick up one foot and work on it comfortably (*right*). This will be the position for treating the soles of the feet. Ask your partner to relax their feet and ankles while you work on them, and let you move them from one position to another without attempting to assist you.

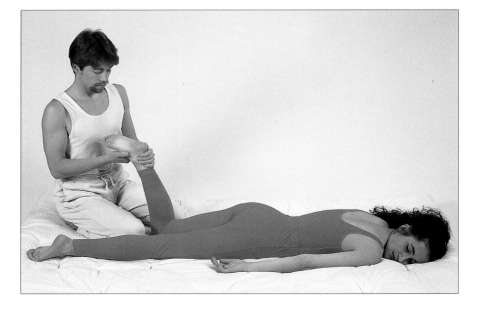

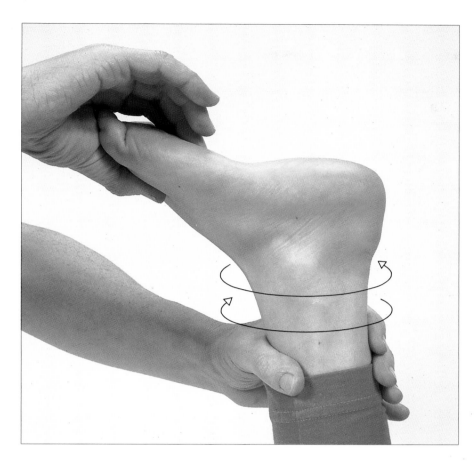

2 Grip the ankle with one hand (*left*), and with the other hand firmly rotate the foot as widely as the ankle will permit. Do this several times in each direction. If you noticed a space under the ankles, when the legs were outstretched, pay attention to them with more rotations.

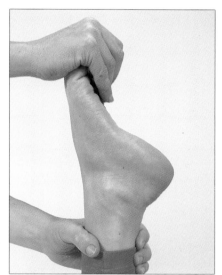

3 Still gripping the ankle, place the palm of your hand over the tops of the toes (*above*), and flex the foot away from you, stretching the whole of the top of the foot, from the ankle down to the tips of the toes. Take the movement to a firm but not painful stretch.

4 Move your passive hand to behind the heel and place the palm of your working hand on the underside of the toes (*left*). Flex the toes downwards forcefully, bringing the stretch into the whole foot, including the Achilles tendon.

These lengthwise flexes are the first two of four overall stretches that can be given to the feet. All can be executed strongly, unless there is a past injury, but should not cause pain. As usual, they are applied on the out-breath, and repeated two or three times; this particular pair can be done with your active arm held straight as in the guidelines.

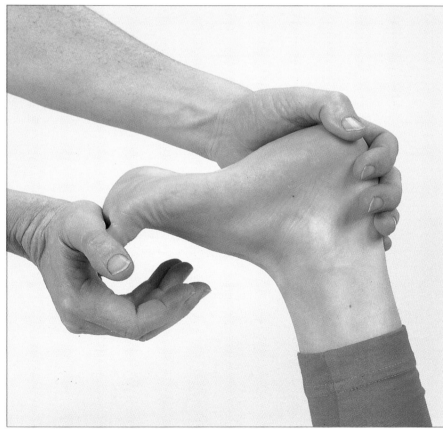

5 With the sole facing away from you, grip each edge of the foot between your fingers and the base of your thumbs, and strongly flex the foot laterally (*right*). Starting with the upper sole and toes, work down to the middle of the foot, repeating the procedure two or three times. This is the first of the two 'crosswise' flexes, which open up Ki flow within the small bones on the top of the feet.

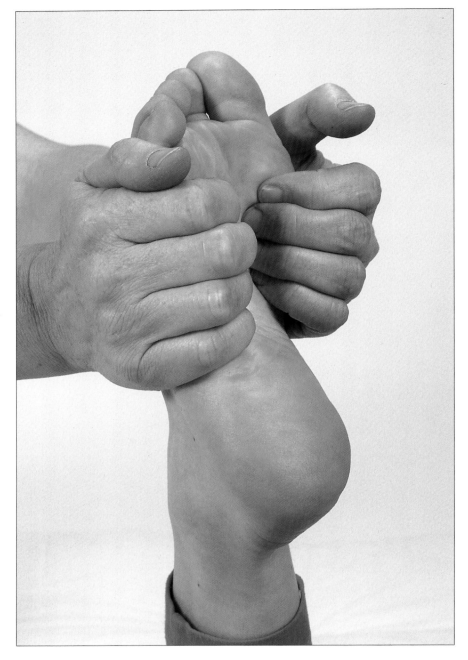

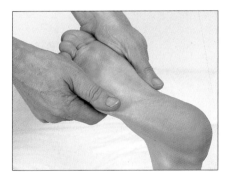

6 Bend the foot from the ankle so that the sole faces upwards. Move your fingers around to the top of the foot and grip the edges again between fingers and base of the thumbs. Flex the foot crosswise downward (*above*), this time opening up the bones in the sole. Move from the upper sole and toes down the length of the sole, almost to the heel.

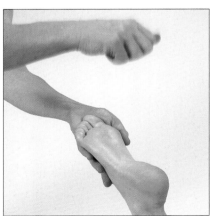

7 Support the foot in one hand and, with the other hand making a loose fist, pound energetically all over the sole (*left*). Keep the wrist relaxed and flexible. You have now loosened up the foot in readiness for the more intense point work to follow.

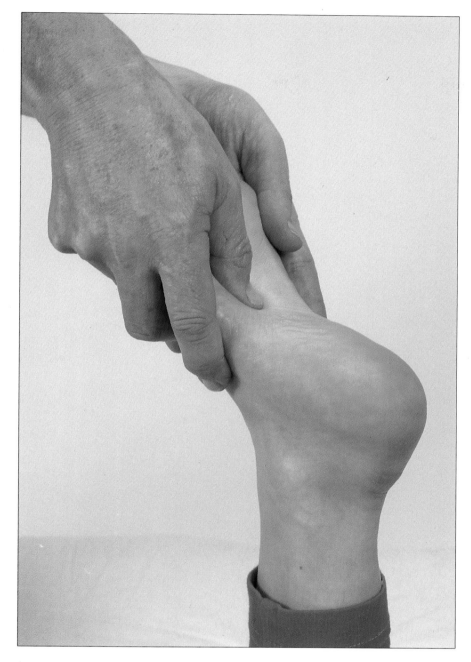

8 Still cradling the foot with one hand, apply thumb pressure over the whole area of the sole of the foot (*left*). As usual, always press in on an out-breath and hold the pressure for a few seconds. First of all, work around the perimeter of the foot: along both edges, round the heel and along the base of the toes. Then press along the centre line, from the base of the toes down to the heel. Some points may be particularly tender, such as those along the instep and in the centre of the upper sole. If so, give them extra treatment, but with lighter pressure. Press more firmly around the harder areas such as the heel and ball of the foot. You cannot use your body weight when working on the sole of the foot, but try to keep the working arm straight while applying thumb pressure.

Soles of the feet pressure points
Lines of treatment for step 8 are shown here (*right*). Press at intervals of about a thumb's width. *Benefits: treatment of these points assists not only the feet, but the whole body, and in particular the kidneys and spleen.*

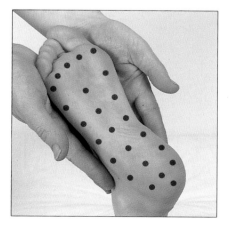

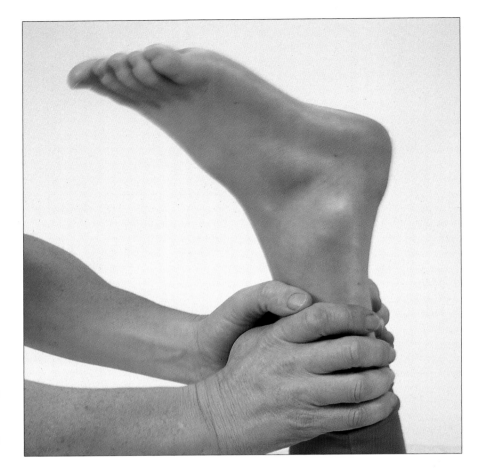

9 To finish this half of the treatment for one foot, grip the ankle with both hands (*right*), and shake the foot vigorously for a few moments. Then move around, position yourself at a comfortable distance from the other foot and repeat steps 2–9.

10 To complete the sequence of the back of the body, which began with lesson 2, stand astride your partner and lightly brush or sweep your hands down the whole of the back of the body (*below*) to enhance the flow of Ki and to finish the section with a light touch and pleasant sensation.

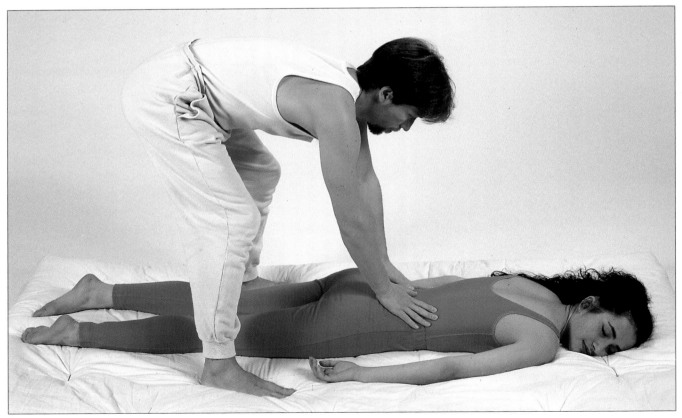

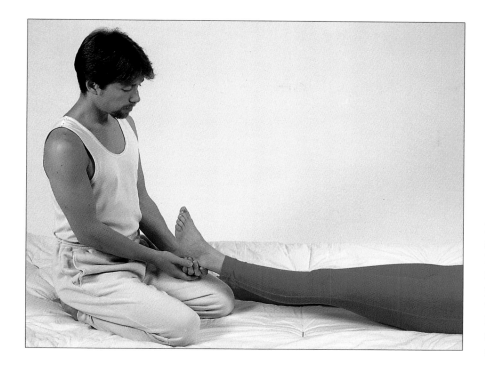

11 Now ask your partner to turn over and lie on their back. Draw the heels downwards to stretch the body, and draw the hands horizontally towards the feet to lower the shoulders. This will be your partner's position for the whole of the rest of the treatment. Kneel or sit below their feet, close enough to hold one foot comfortably in your hands (*left*).

12 With your passive hand supporting the foot, apply thumb pressure to the top of the foot (*left*), along each of the channels that run between the bones there, starting between the toes and working up into the ankle. Pay special attention to points that feel especially tender to your partner, by working lightly but repeatedly over them.

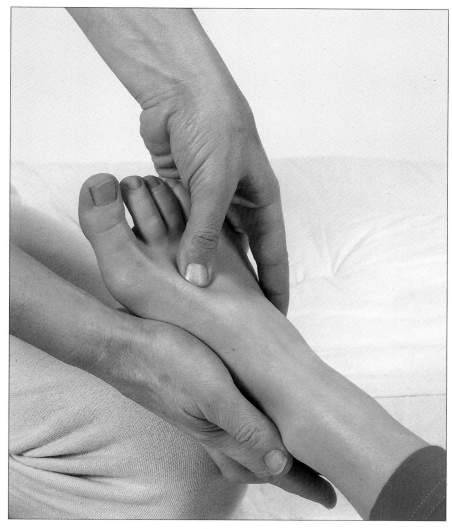

Top of the foot pressure points
The points used in step 12 occur in lines along the top of the foot (*below*), in channels between the bones that run from toes to ankles. Press at intervals of a thumb's width, as usual.
Benefits: helpful to the liver, the stomach and the gall bladder.

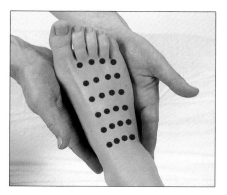

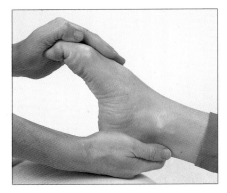

13 The remainder of the foot treatment focuses on the toes. Support the heel with your passive hand, lay the fingers of your other hand over the tops of the toes and flex them firmly downwards with the heels of your palms (*right*).

14 Now rest the heel of your working hand against the underside of the toes and wrap your fingers around them. Flex the toes strongly, all together, in the opposite direction to that in the previous step (*right*).

Treating the toes is helpful for the organs that connect with them: the liver, the gall bladder, the spleen, the stomach and the bladder.

15 Resting the foot on your knee, grip it just below the base of the big toe, and with your previously passive hand hold that toe between forefinger and thumb. Now rotate the toe firmly in wide circles, three times in each direction. Continue working on this toe for the following three steps: 16–18.

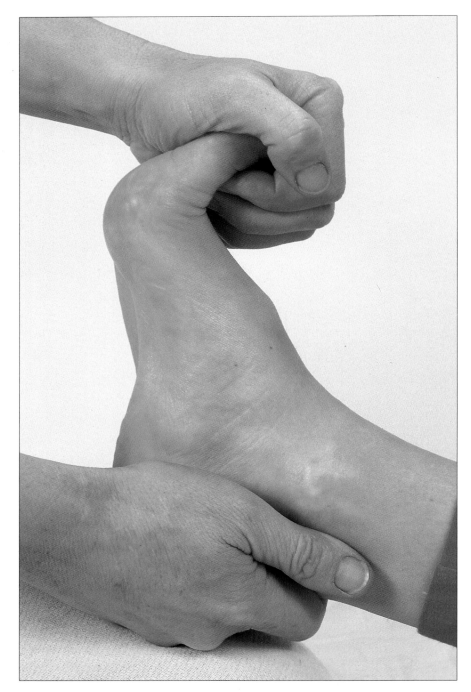

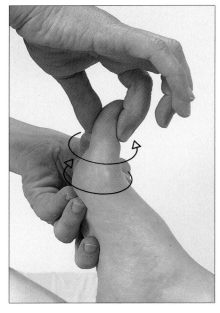

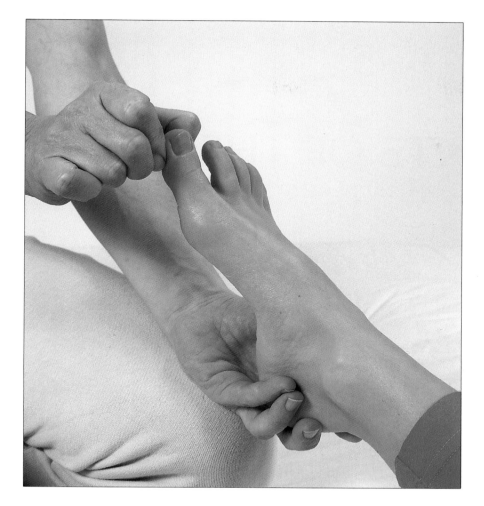

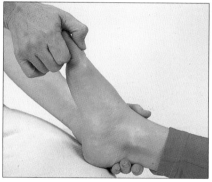

16 Lower your supporting hand to the ankle, and squeeze the big toe firmly, with your thumb on top and your curled forefinger underneath (*above*). Move from the base of the toe up to the nail, pressing in with the tip of your thumb.

17 Now grip the end of the toe on either side (*left*), and pinch strongly a couple of times on the soft portion at the tip of the toe, above the nail.

18 To finish the treatment of this toe, grip the foot around the ankle again, and pull the toe firmly towards you with the thumb on the top of the foot and the fingers underneath. Start at the root of the toe and then pull from the other two joints. Repeat steps 15–18 for each of the other toes in turn.

Then move on to the other foot, turn back to page 51 and repeat steps 11–18. While treating the toes, remember that some people are very sensitive about them being touched; they may feel ticklish to a light touch, but would respond better to firm treatment, while others genuinely feel vulnerable and can only take gentle work. Regular treatment of the feet can actually help overcome these problems of sensitivity.

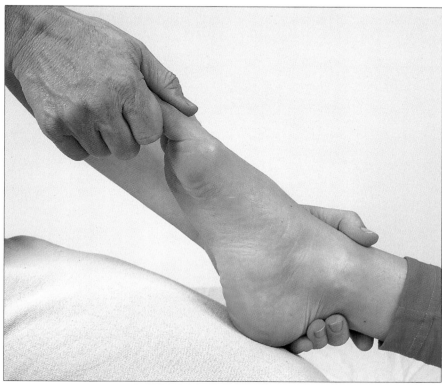

5

THE FRONTS OF THE LEGS

Many of the points that were made about the legs in lesson 3 also apply here. Like the backs of the legs, work on the fronts helps to promote a feeling of groundedness, encouraging awareness lower down in the body, rather than in the head – a common problem in modern society. Work here also helps to stimulate Ki, or energy flow in the legs. This helps to combat deterioration of general health caused by lack of vitality in the legs due to a sedentary lifestyle.

There are one or two aspects that particularly concern the fronts of the legs, and the pelvic area, which also receives treatment in this lesson. They represent a person's attitude to the future: they literally face ahead, and are concerned with 'moving forward' in life on both an actual and on a psychological level.

Thinking ahead is an issue for many people, and treatment here may well both highlight this as a problem area and, over a period, move energy in a way that enables progress at an emotional level. The inner thighs and the pelvis in particular are sexually significant; tension or vulnerability here can indicate this. Treatment can be beneficial, but if there is sensitivity avoid excessive pressure.

About this sequence
The treatment begins with overall rotations and stretches, moving on to palming, and then pressure-point work on one leg and then the other. The front and inner surfaces of the legs carry the channels for the kidneys, spleen and pancreas, liver and stomach, so treatment will particularly benefit these organs.

1 Your partner will be lying flat on their back, following the feet sequence. Move from your sitting or kneeling position to stand astride your partner's ankles; pick up their legs behind the knees, so that the knees bend, and place the feet flat on the floor (right). Place your hands on the knees, and push them away from you, so that the feet leave the floor.

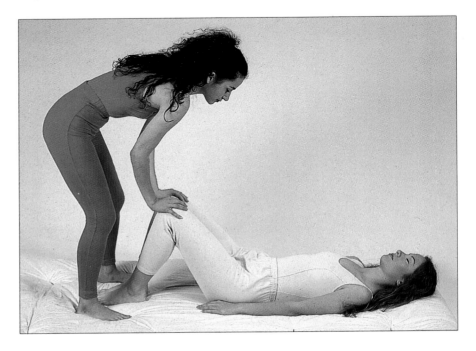

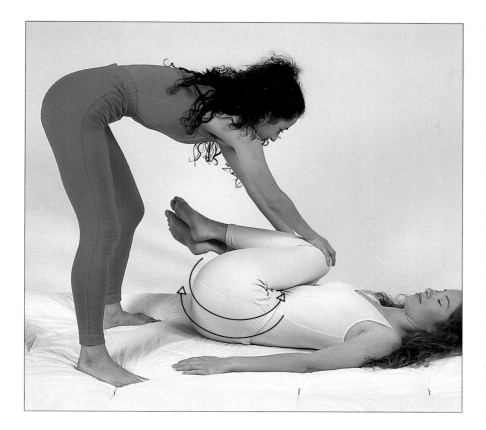

2 Rotate the legs in a wide circle, keeping the knees together (*left*). Ask your partner to relax their legs; they will feel heavy, so be prepared for this. Make sure you are focusing attention in your abdomen; this helps to keep you balanced. Rotate the legs three times in each direction, or more if the knees or hips seem stiff. The state of the knees reflects the condition of the organs you are working on in this sequence – the kidneys, spleen, pancreas, liver and stomach.

3 Using your own body weight, lean in and press the knees firmly towards the chest (*left*). Hold the position for the full out-breath, release for the in-breath, and stretch again two more times. Apply the stretch to a degree that suits your partner, just until you begin to feel resistance; it should not be a painful stretch. Then guide the feet back down on to the floor, into the starting position on the opposite page.

These rotations and stretches help open up the hip and knee joints and the lower back; they are particularly helpful where there is stiffness or lack of flexibility in these areas. In addition, they encourage useful overall Ki movement through the whole lower body, before you begin to treat the legs individually.

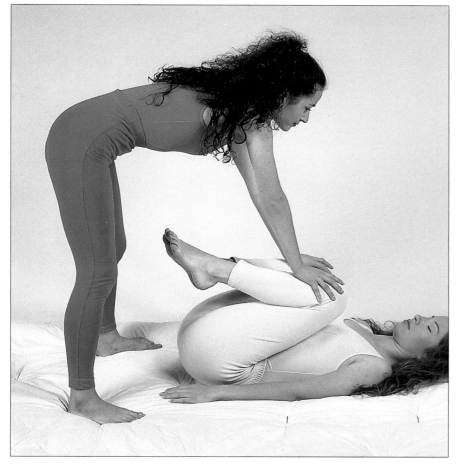

4 Move into the 'lunge' position with your front foot alongside your partner's hip. Place one hand on the knee, and pick up the foot by the heel (*right*). You will be working with this leg until the end of the sequence, when you will begin again from this step with the other leg. Ask your partner to relax and not control the leg at all; then take it in wide rotations, allowing it to fall sideways to its natural limit, especially outwards away from the hip and over towards the other leg (*below*). Rotate the leg slowly three times in each direction. Maintain this hold on the leg for the next step.

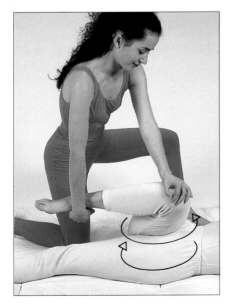

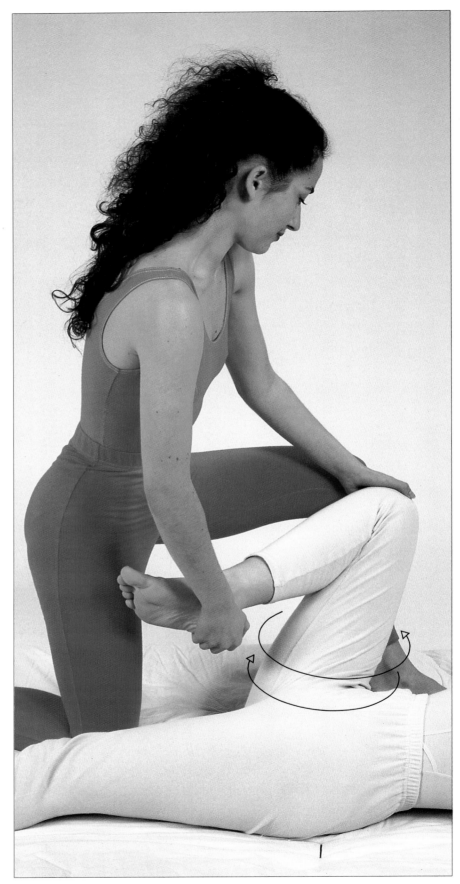

CAUTION

Do not use this stretch on the elderly, or where there is an injury or arthritis in the knee or hip joints. Work gently if the hip or knee are very stiff.

5 With your hand on the front of the knee, lean forward to stretch the leg in towards the chest. As usual, apply the stretch and hold for the out-breath, release for an in-breath and repeat this two more times. Continue to hold the leg for the next step.

6 Remaining in the same position, place your partner's foot on the far side of their opposite leg (*right*). Place one hand on the knee, and the other hand on the shoulder (*below*). By bringing your weight forward over the body, pushing the knee towards the floor, you can exert a powerful cross-stretch. Repeat three times with the out-breaths; you will find that the stretch naturally goes a little further each time. If you are unsure about how much pressure to exert, check with your partner that it is comfortable and not too strong.

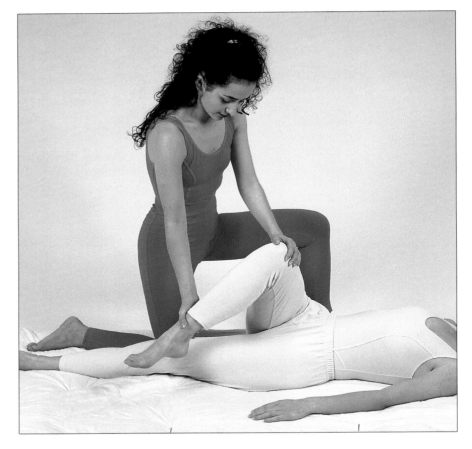

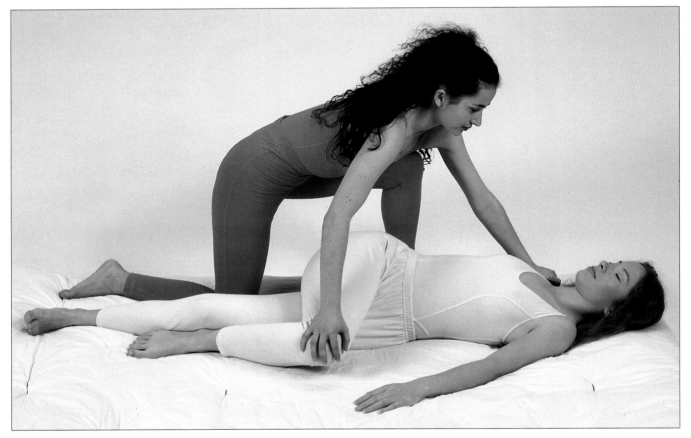

7 Bring your partner's leg back towards you, place the foot on the floor beside the knee of the stationary leg, and let the other knee drop down towards the floor. Place one hand on your partner's hip and the other on the opposite knee (*below*), and exert a gentle stretch to open up the hip. Do not use all of your weight here: this is a much gentler stretch than the previous one. Stay on the same side of the body, to continue work on this leg.

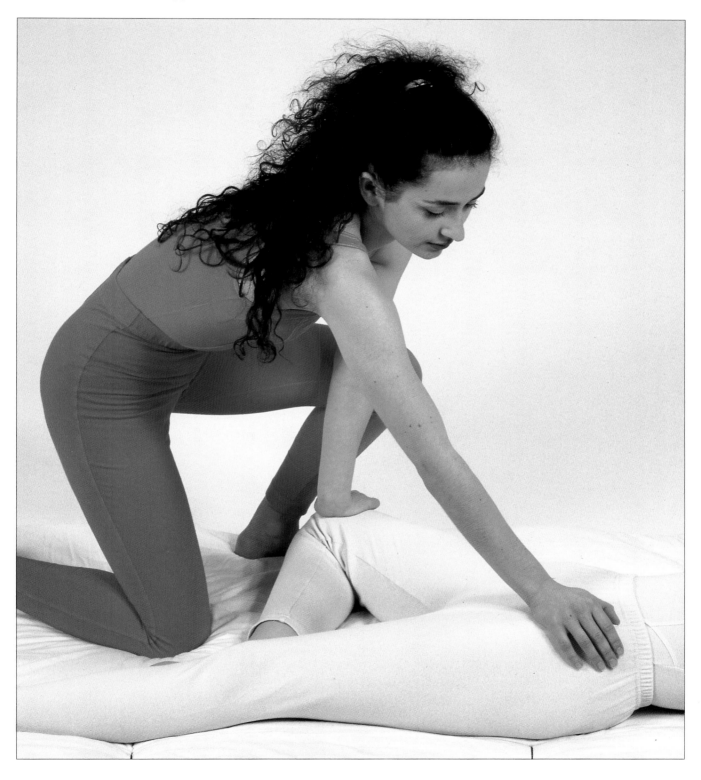

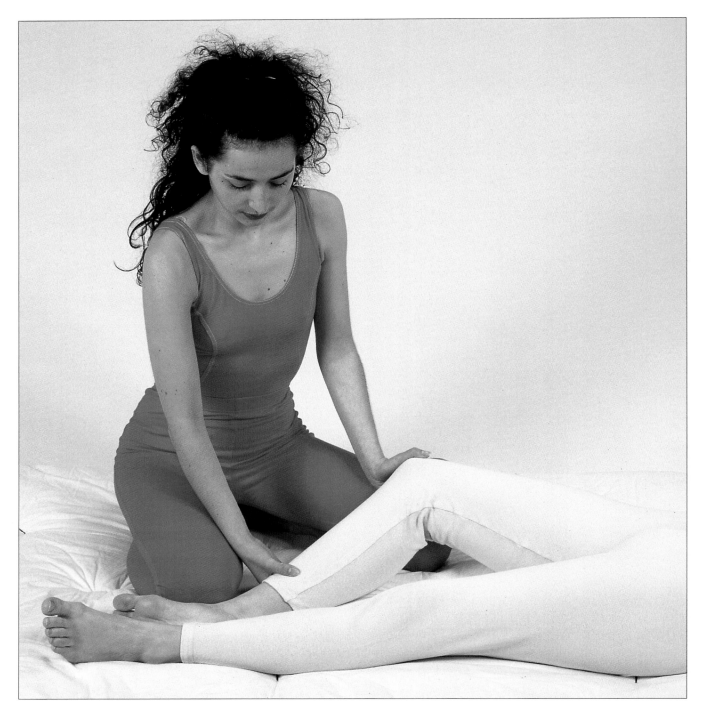

8 Adopt a kneeling position
alongside your partner's lower
leg, with your knees spread
apart for balance and your body
facing theirs at a slight angle
(*above*). Draw the foot up a little
until the heel is opposite the ankle-
bone on the other foot (*right*). You
should sit close enough to your

partner so that you can rest their
raised knee on your own knee;
but before you give support, let
the knee drop to its natural level,
and then slide your knee under
to provide support at this height.
This will prevent strain on the hip
or knee joints when you apply
palm and thumb pressure.

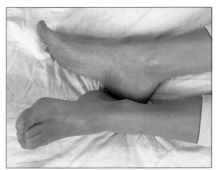

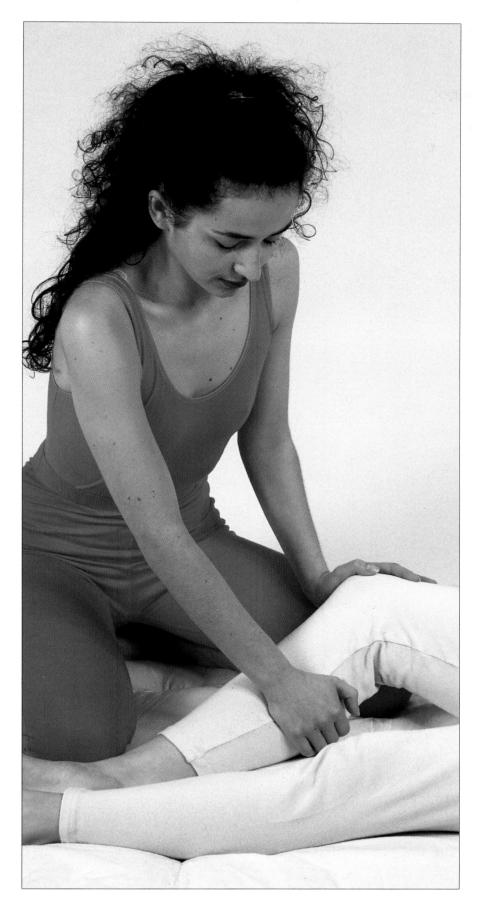

CAUTION

Do not treat the lower leg during pregnancy.

9 Apply palm pressure from the ankle up to the knee, avoiding direct pressure on the knee, leaning in with the heel of the palm between the shin-bone and the calf muscle. Have the passive hand on the kneecap. Palm along this line three times in total, exerting pressure on the out-breath. Notice whether there are any points that feel blocked.

Then palm up the centre line of the inside of the thigh (*below*). The guideline is to work along the large muscle that you will be able to feel under the surface when the leg is in this slightly-stretched position. Repeat twice more.

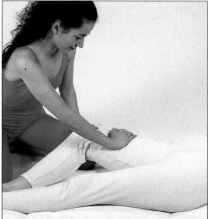

10 Apply thumb pressure along the same line (*right*), pressing in against the underside of the shin-bone, from the ankle up to the knee. Some of these points may be very tender, particularly just above the ankle and just below the knee; if so, treat more times but with less pressure.

Then start again above the knee, re-positioning the passive hand on top of the thigh, and proceed along the centre line of the inner thigh up towards the groin (*right*). Stop short of the genital area, in order to avoid embarrassment. As with the palming, your guideline is to work along the centre of the large muscle that comes up in this position. Repeat the whole series of points two more times.

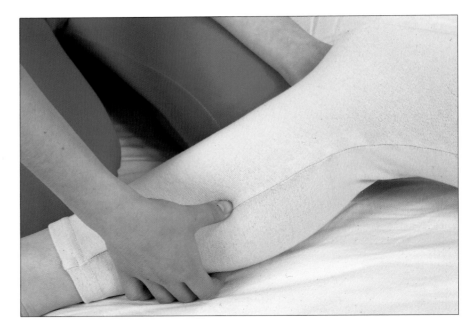

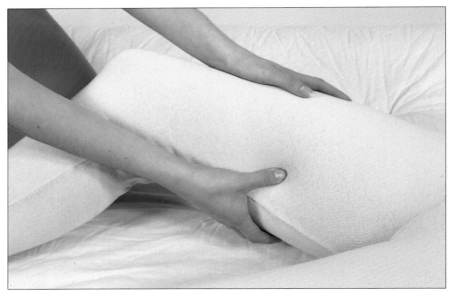

Inner leg pressure points: first line
These points occur in a line between the shin-bone and calf muscle on the lower leg and continue up the inside of the thigh (*right*). Treat the points, as usual, at intervals of about one thumb width, starting above the ankle and missing out the knee.
Benefits: particularly helpful for the spleen.

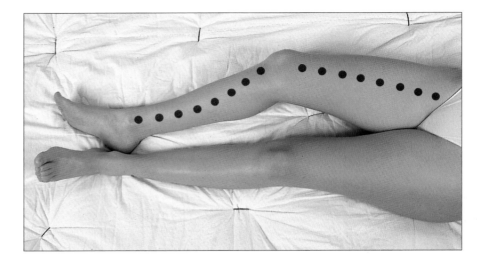

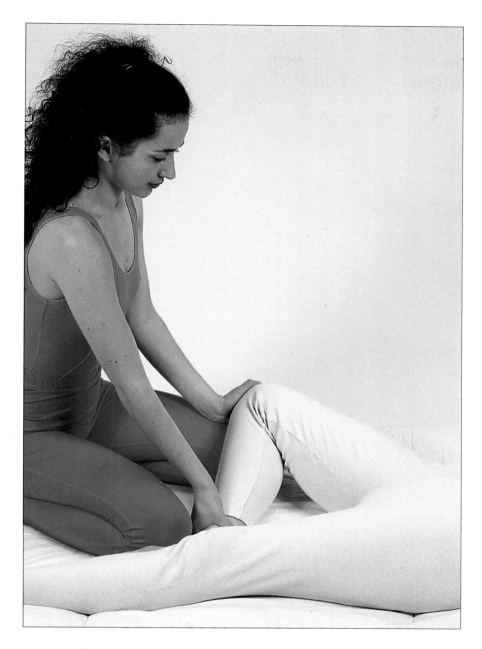

11 Rotate your position slightly, and bring your partner's foot higher up until the instep is opposite the knee (*below*). As before, let the knee drop to its natural unsupported position, and then bring your knee in underneath to support it at this height. Again place the passive hand on the kneecap (*left*).

Do palm work from the ankle to the knee, along the line of points shown (*bottom left*) and then from the knee to the groin; in the thigh section, you can again work along the large muscle, which has been brought to a new position relative to the surface channels by moving the angle of the leg. Repeat the palm work twice more.

Then continue with thumb work along the same line as before, working over the line three times in each case.

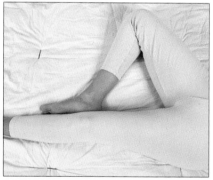

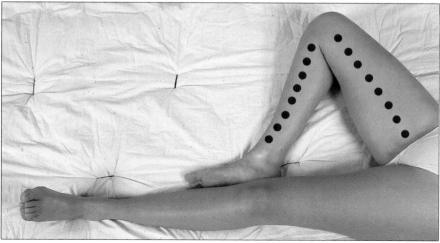

Inner leg pressure points: second line

The second line of inner leg points (*left*) are treated with the leg in this position. Treat the points as usual at intervals of about one thumb's width, missing out the knee. For many people, the inner thigh points may feel very tight and feel quite painful. If so, work gently but with more repetition.

Benefits: these points assist the liver in particular.

63

12 Rotate your body a little more, and bring your partner's foot higher still, towards the groin (*below*). As before, let the knee drop to its natural unsupported position, and then bring your knee in underneath to support it at this height (*right*).

Palm from the ankle to the knee and then from the knee to the groin; as before, over the thigh section, you can again work along the large muscle that appears. Follow this with thumb pressure-point work along the same line (*bottom right*). Carry out both procedures three times.

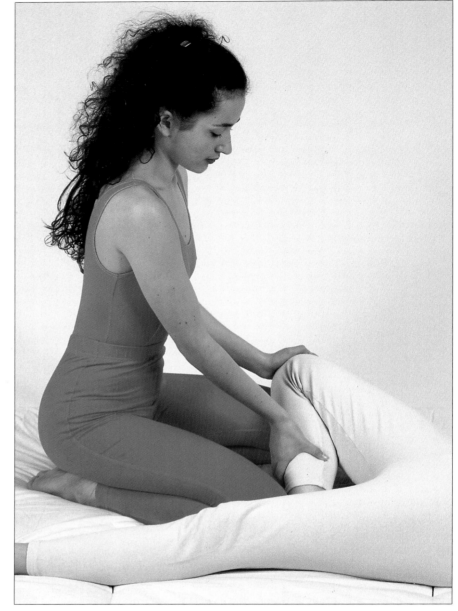

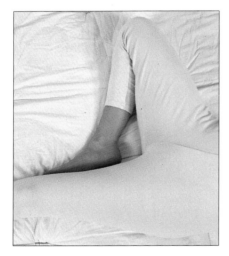

Inner leg pressure points: third line
To treat this line of points, the foot should be as near to the groin as it will comfortably go (*right*). Treat the points again at intervals of about one thumb's width, missing out the area over the knee.
Benefits: treating these points particularly helps the kidneys.

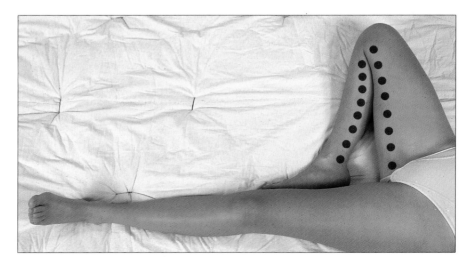

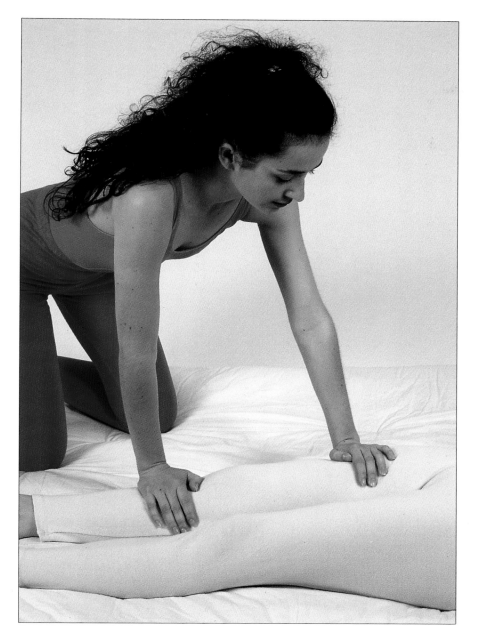

CAUTION

*Do not treat the lower leg
during pregnancy.*

13 Straighten out your partner's leg, and come up on all fours opposite their knees. Keeping one hand just below the knee, palm with the other hand along the front of the thigh, just on the near side of the centre line (*left*). This time you start at the top of the thigh and work down to the knee. Then move the passive hand down to the foot (*bottom left*) and continue palming from the knee to the ankle, again just to your side of the centre line: in the channel between the front of the shin-bone and the outer muscles. The line to follow is shown at the bottom of the following page.

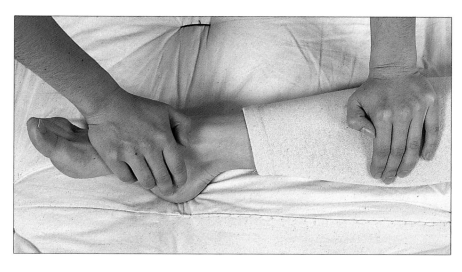

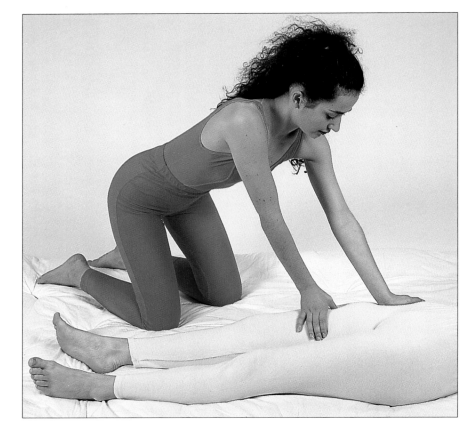

14 Turn yourself slightly towards your partner's upper body and place one hand on your partner's hip (*right*). With the other hand, apply thumb pressure along the line you have just palmed. Some people are rather ticklish in this area, so be aware of your partner's reaction. When you come to the knee, rotate your body back again to face the lower leg and apply thumb pressure on the lower section (*right*), avoiding the knee itself.

This completes the treatment of the first leg. Now turn back to page 56 go to your partner's other side, and repeat steps 4–13 on the other leg.

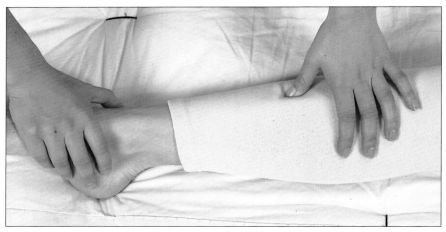

Front of leg pressure points
Notice that the direction of work for these points (*right*) is from thigh to ankle, the opposite to that in the last three cases. As always, apply thumb pressure at intervals of a thumb width.
Benefits: treatment of these points particularly helps the stomach.

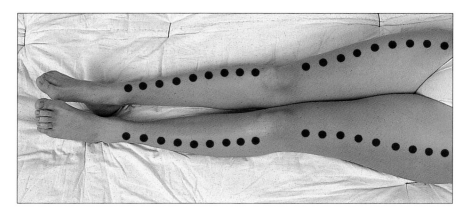

15 To complete the treatment of the legs, brush with your fingertips from the toes up to the hips (*below*). This stimulatets the flow of energy in the legs, bringing a feeling of unity after the more detailed pressure-point work. It also completes work on the legs with a gentle sensation. You are now ready to treat the abdomen.

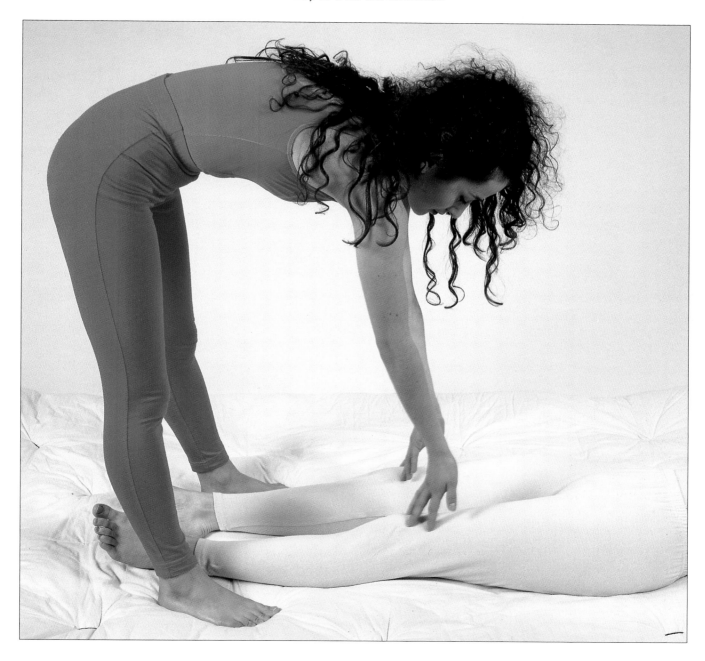

6

THE ABDOMEN

For the purpose of treatment in this lesson, the abdomen means the soft, malleable area below the ribs and above the pelvis and pubic bone. This area contains unprotected and partially protected vital organs – the liver, gall bladder, stomach, spleen and pancreas, all partly under the ribs; then, below that, the large intestine or colon, surrounding the small intestine, with the kidneys behind; and lower still, the bladder and reproductive organs (see page 126). Treatment must take into account the vulnerability of these organs, and pressure should be modified accordingly if there is a known problem with any of them, or if any treatment causes sharp or sudden pain.

The abdomen is sensitive or tense in some people; watch your partner's face from time to time as you work on it, or check by asking them, and temper the pressure if you observe discomfort. Pent-up emotions are often held in the abdomen, rather than being outwardly expressed, causing sensitivity here. The following treatment can help release them.

The abdomen, called the 'hara' in Japanese, contains an important internal energy centre, the Tan Den, in the middle of its lower half. This is considered in the Orient to be the major centre of the body's underlying energy and strength. Its condition profoundly affects general health, vitality and longevity. If the hara is healthy, you will find a sense of strong energy here; it should seem bouncy and resilient to the touch; not hard, excessively swollen or, on the other hand, completely soft and lifeless.

The upper half of the abdominal cavity should feel reasonably soft and open. Hardness and impenetrability here is a reflection of the underlying condition of the organs beneath, indicating stagnation or imbalances in Ki flow. This part of the abdomen also houses the solar plexus centre, which governs issues of confidence and exercise of will power. Tension in this area, particularly in the diaphragm, also reflects pent-up emotion, often related to these issues. Shiatsu helps with release of these tensions, and over a period can profoundly support this aspect of personal development.

About this sequence

This sequence begins with 'tuning in' to the hara, before the preparatory massage work to loosen up the area, and finishes with specific point work. Massage and pressure-point work on the abdomen directly affect the functioning of both the small and large intestines. The abdomen mirrors the condition of the whole person, and comprehensive treatment here will help restore Ki imbalances. Working on the abdomen can be most profound.

POINTS TO REMEMBER

- *use your body weight, not muscular effort*
- *keep your own body relaxed*
- *focus attention and breathe in your abdomen*
- *keep your working arm straight but not locked*
- *lean into each movement on the out-breath, and hold the position*
- *work at right angles to the body surface*
- *cultivate a calm feeling and regular rhythm*

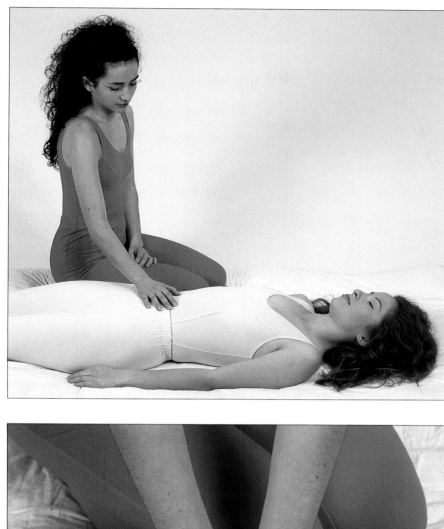

1 Kneel alongside your partner, close enough to be able to lay one hand on the abdomen and still keep your own back straight without feeling overbalanced (*left*). Keep your hand here for a few moments, making a connection with your partner's Ki and cultivating a calm and peaceful feeling, before starting the treatment.

If your partner's abdomen has been troublesome, for instance with severe constipation or diarrhoea, they may find it helpful to draw the knees up and place the feet flat on the floor instead of having the legs straight.

2 Begin to massage across the abdominal area with both hands. Start with your hands at the side nearest to you, positioned close to the ribs, and push gently down and across with the heels of your hands (*left*); then pull your hands back towards you (*below*), pressing down and in with the fingers. Continue these movements in a slow but smoothly connected action, not unlike the kneading of bread dough. Gradually press more firmly and deeply, covering the whole area between the ribs and the pubic bone.

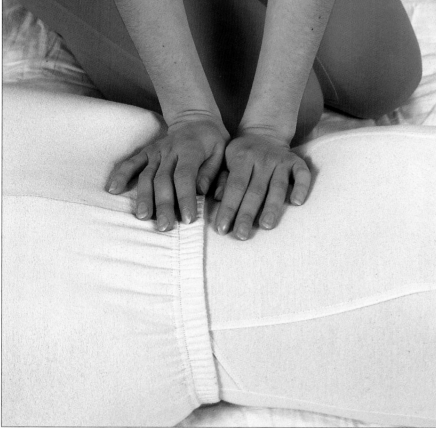

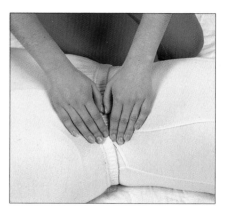

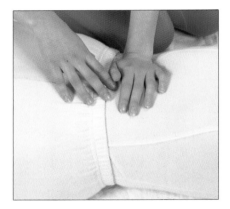

3 Starting with the lower area of your partner's abdomen on the side nearest you, apply palm pressure downwards, and continue in a circular direction, clockwise around the navel (*above*). Keep the passive hand resting on the hip at first, while you move around with the other hand, making particularly sure that you exert pressure on the out-breath. The area of treatment is shown at the bottom of the opposite page. When you are about halfway round, you will find it more comfortable and effective to rest the working hand and continue with what was the passive hand (*right*) to complete the circle. Start with light pressure, and then repeat twice more, leaning in with increasing pressure each time; you can generally work quite strongly in this area, but do check your partner's reaction.

CAUTION

Do not work here during advanced pregnancy. Work more lightly during menstruation, or in cases of abdominal or reproductive organ problems.

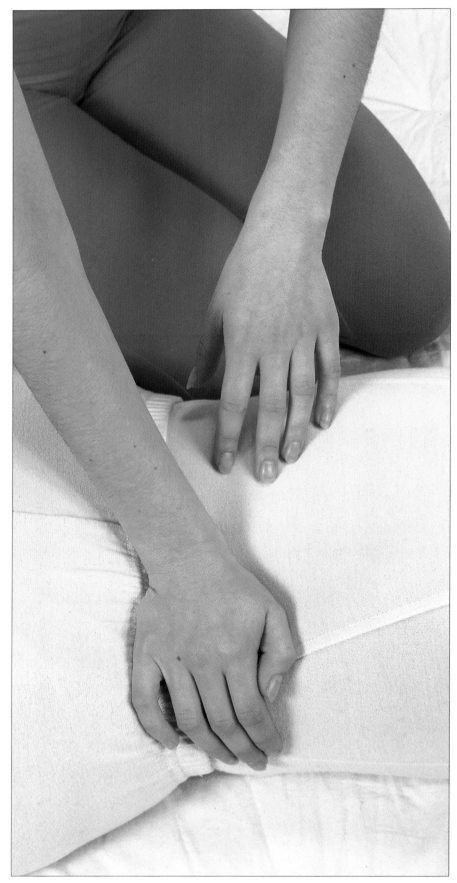

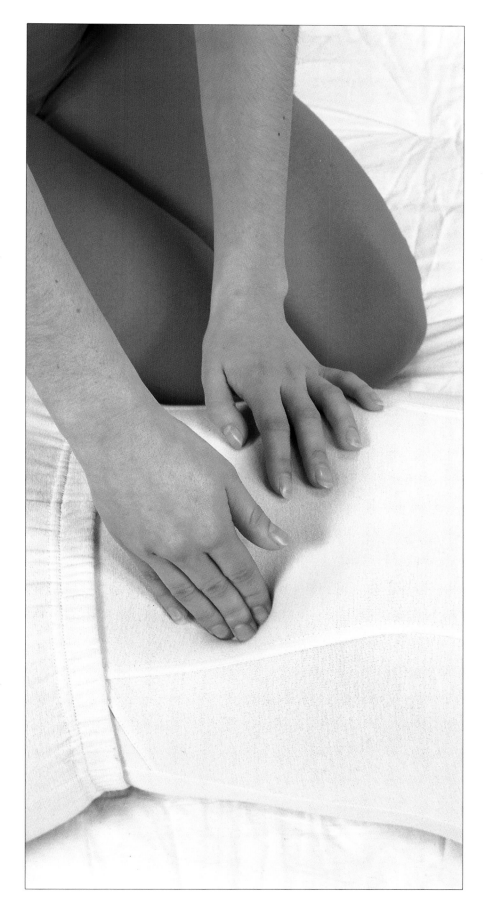

4 Now proceed with more localized point work over the same area; again starting near the hip on your side and working in a clockwise direction, applying pressure on the out-breath. However, instead of using thumb pressure, you can use the tips of the fingers (*left*). Hold the fingers straight and close together and press inwards, perpendicular to the skin's surface. The hands will alternate roles, between passive and working, as in the previous step. Repeat twice more.

Finish by placing your hands one on top of the other, and go over the same area again, sliding your hands in a clockwise direction, to complete work on the abdomen.

Abdominal pressure points

The approximate line to work around forms a circle about 5 centimetres (2 inches) out from the navel, depending on your partner's size. If you find points that seem hard, or feel tender to your partner, press more lightly but repeatedly. If there is sharp pain, leave that spot immediately.

Benefits: useful for all the abdominal organs; helpful for constipation, cramps, poor digestion, pre-menstrual tension and other menstrual problems, urination difficulties, lack of sexual energy and overall vitality.

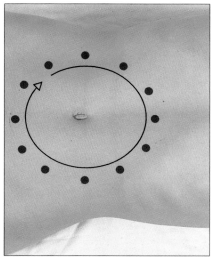

7

THE HANDS

Having evolved from feet, human hands still bear a structural similarity to them – many small bones forming the body of the hand, and with fingers analogous to toes but more elongated and articulate. So, treatment of hands is very similar to that used for the feet.

The hands have developed to enable us to carry out more intricate tasks; they are the tools we use for fixing and making things. It follows that when the hands are not functioning as they should, and you cannot 'do things', it may be that you just need a rest. Our society tends to be focused on constantly 'having something to do'. This tendency for hands to be active means that when they passively receive treatment, it can be a surprisingly profound and even sensuous experience.

In the Orient, people have long realized the value of hand massage. All over the East you can see traders haggling over prices, automatically massaging their own hands to prevent the nervousness that would perhaps spoil a deal. Likewise, even in Western society, people instinctively wring their hands to help deal with shock, worry or grief.

About this sequence

As with the feet, the treatment sequence starts with overall loosening and flexing before going into detailed work on points and then treating the fingers, for each hand in turn. Like the feet, the hands are rich in nerve endings, and half the energy channels begin or end here. The connection with heart and circulation is particularly strong, but hand treatment can benefit the whole system.

1 The whole of this sequence is carried out on each hand in turn, so when you reach the end of the sequence with one hand, go back to the beginning and treat the other hand. Position yourself to one side of your partner; you will be treating the hand on that side from now on. Grip their wrist with one hand, and hold the middle of the hand between the thumb and fingers of your other hand (*right*). Firmly rotate the hand three times in each direction, flexing the wrist as far as it will comfortably go in every direction. Keep hold of that wrist for the next step.

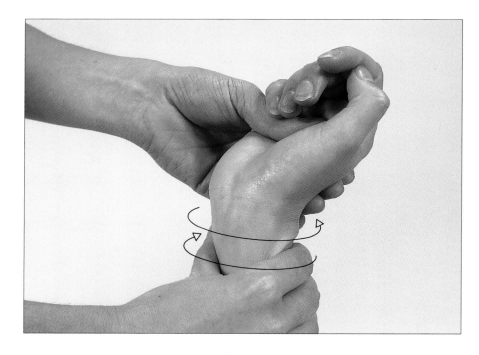

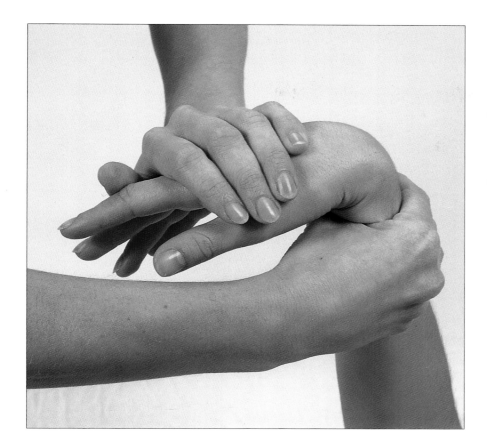

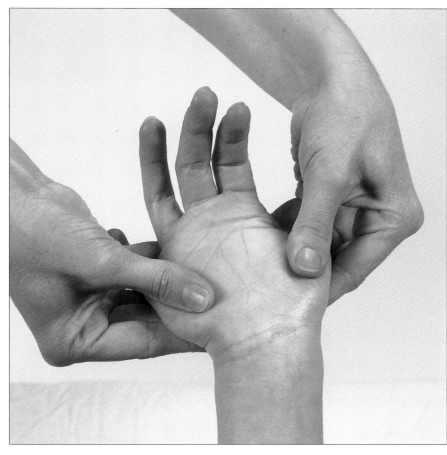

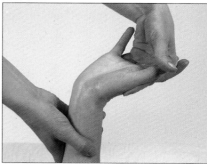

2 Interlink the fingers of your working hand with your partner's, and flex the hand firmly backwards (*above*), adjusting the grip with your passive hand to a more comfortable one. Stretch only as far as the wrist will naturally go. Hold for the out-breath. Repeat twice more.

3 Return to the original grip and flex your partner's hand downwards (*left*) from above with the palm of your hand. Repeat twice more.

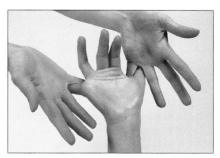

4 Turn your partner's palm upwards and thread your little fingers under their thumb and little finger respectively (*above*). Place your thumbs at the edges of the palm (*left*) and press downwards flexing the palm open. Repeat for two more out-breaths.

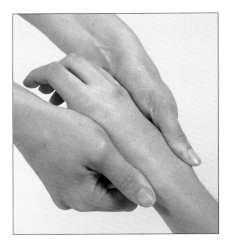

5 Now turn the palm over and grip the edges of the hand between your fingers and the base of your thumbs (*right*). Pressing down and moving outwards across the top of the hand with your thumbs, flex the hand downwards three times on the out-breaths.

6 Turn the hand palm upwards again, and apply thumb pressure over the whole of the palm (*right*). Cover the perimeter of the palm, the base of the thumb and the centre of the palm, applying pressure on the out-breaths, as usual. You can work strongly into these points.

Palm pressure points
Approximate lines of treatment run down between the bones in the hand (*below*). Pay special attention to areas that seem hard or tight, working repeatedly over them. *Benefits: helpful for stiffness or arthritis in the hands; also benefits the heart, circulation and energy levels, plus the lungs and breathing.*

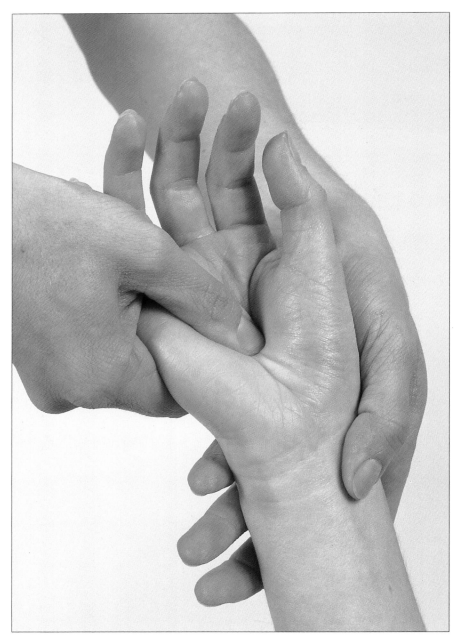

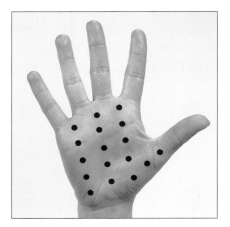

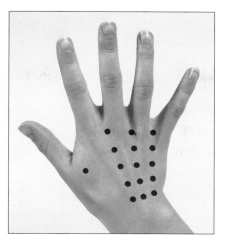

7 Turn the hand over again and, holding the wrist with the passive hand, apply thumb pressure to the back of the hand (*below*). Work from between each of the fingers, along the channels that lie between the bones, up into the wrist.

Back of the hand pressure points
Lines of treatment are between the bones (*left*). As usual, work at intervals of a thumb's width.
Benefits: helpful for circulation and arthritis in the hands; also benefits the large and small intestines, and body metabolism in general.

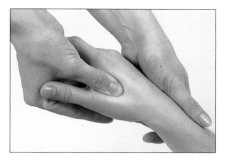

8 Move your hand in between your partner's thumb and forefinger (*above*), with your thumb on top and your forefinger underneath. Press strongly into the web of skin just beyond the muscle that you find there. Repeat twice.

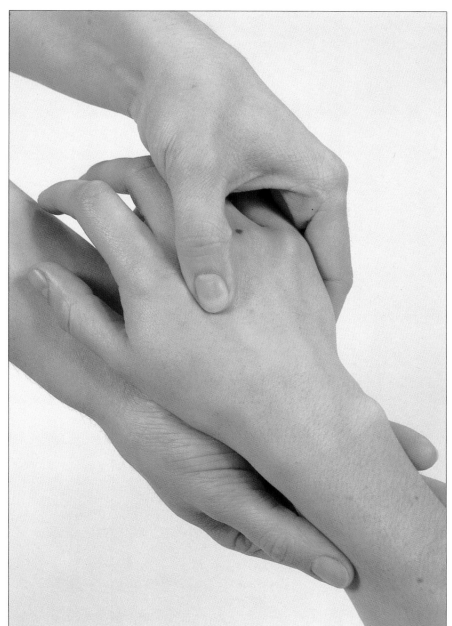

CAUTION

Do not apply pressure between thumb and forefinger (above) *during pregnancy*

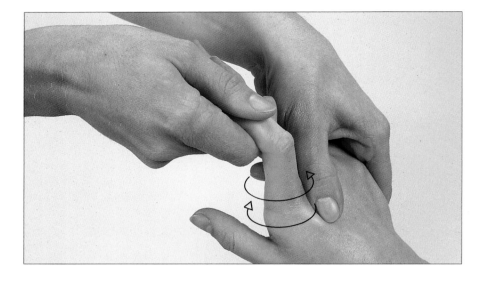

9 With your passive hand, grip your partner's hand just below the base of the forefinger. With the other hand, grip the forefinger above the middle joint with your thumb on top (*right*), and firmly rotate it three times in each direction. Keep hold of this finger for the next step.

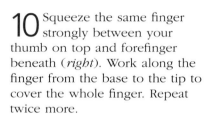

10 Squeeze the same finger strongly between your thumb on top and forefinger beneath (*right*). Work along the finger from the base to the tip to cover the whole finger. Repeat twice more.

11 Still supporting the hand, keep working on this finger. This time, turn your hand slightly sideways and strongly pinch the soft part of the tip of the finger, on either side of the nail, between your thumb and forefinger (*right*). Repeat twice more.

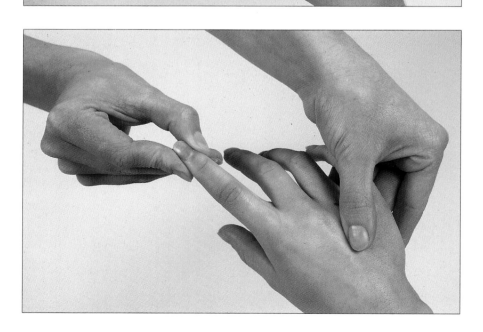

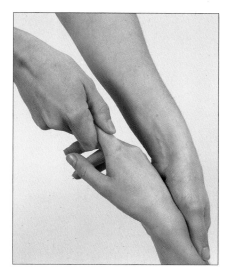

12 Turn your hand back again, so that the tip of your thumb is on top of the finger, and grip it just above the root (*left*) gripping the wrist with your other hand, and pull the finger strongly towards you, on an out-breath. Then let your grip of the finger slide out to the second section, or phalange, and pull again from just above the knuckle. Finally do the same with the end section, pulling from the tip.

Take each of the other fingers in turn, as well as the thumb, and repeat steps 9–12.

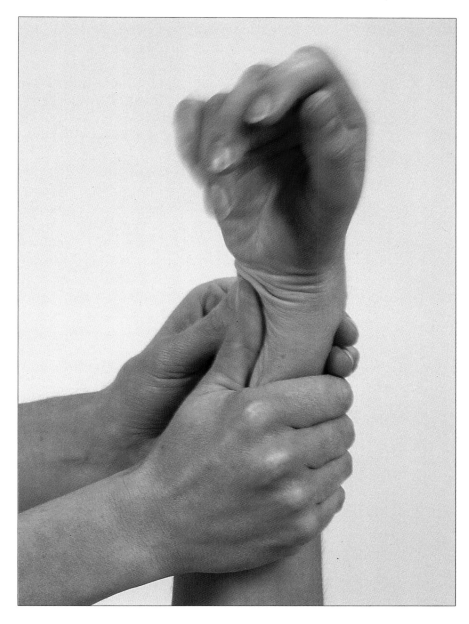

13 Grip the wrist with both your hands and shake it vigorously for a few moments, to disperse the energy in the points you have been treating and to complete the treatment of this hand.

Now turn back to page 72, move to your partner's opposite side, and repeat steps 1–13 for the other hand. Stay on that side for the treatment of the arm.

8

THE ARMS

As the hands were once feet, so the arms were once another set of legs at a time when our ancestors walked on all fours. This means that there is an underlying analogy with the legs, and this reflects in patterns of Ki flow and the Shiatsu approach to treatment. As with the legs, six of the classical energy meridians travel through the arms; half of these begin in the hands and run on the back of the arms, and half run on the front surfaces ending in the hands, in a similar way to the meridians in the legs, with opposite directions of 'flow' on each surface.

The arms are closely associated with two major internal energy centres in the upper thorax – the heart and throat chakras. These each affect and reflect their own set of life issues: the heart centre is especially concerned with the emotions, emotional aspects of relationships, the ability to be compassionate and emotional responses to life events; the throat chakra relates to communication. Problems in any of these areas of life will often show up in the arms, and treatment, over a period of time, can help with these matters. Along with the hands, the arms are also more specifically associated with the heart and circulation. Likewise, the condition of the arms generally reflects that of the chest. The elbows are concerned with the body's middle organs: the liver and gall bladder, and the stomach and spleen. The wrists are associated with the condition of the kidneys and the reproductive organs.

Now that we walk in an upright fashion, the arms, no longer having to bear the body weight, have evolved in a specialized direction. Like the hands, they too are now agents of doing, with the added symbolic component of reaching out to other people. Together with the hands, they are also our agents for giving and receiving, as well as for gesticulation and physical expression. So all these personal issues, too, can show up in the arms. In many people, the arms are not used to being in a passive state and receiving treatment; this can show as an inability to relax and relinquish. If you find this happening, just give more treatment, especially preparatory stretches and release work.

About this sequence
The sequence begins with preparatory rotations and stretches, followed by palming and thumbing for each surface of the arm in turn. Treatment of the arms is directly helpful for physical problems such as tennis elbow, long-term injuries, general stiffness, aches and pains, as well as complex ailments like arthritis. There is also benefit for the organs whose channels run through the arms – the heart, the intestines, as well as the lungs and breathing, circulation and metabolism in general.

POINTS TO REMEMBER

- *use your body weight, not muscular effort*
- *keep your own body relaxed*
- *focus attention and breathe in your abdomen*
- *keep your working arm straight but not locked*
- *lean into each movement on the out-breath, and hold the position*
- *work at right angles to the body surface*
- *cultivate a calm feeling and regular rhythm*

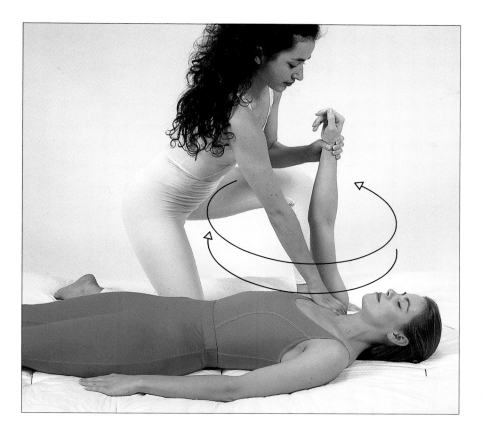

1 In this sequence, again, you will complete the treatment on one arm, then move to the other and carry out the same routine there. Adopt the lunge position alongside your partner, putting your front foot level with their shoulder. Place your hand on their shoulder, and grip their wrist with your other hand (*left*). Holding the shoulder in place, make circles as large as possible with the arm, three times in each direction, to free energy through the shoulder joint and into the arm. Keep holding both wrist and shoulder throughout.

Then, lunge forward on an out-breath, still holding the shoulder, and stretch the arm backwards (*below*). Use your whole body to do this. Release for an in-breath, and stretch again, twice. If there is arthritis or any other weakness in the arm, or if the shoulder is stiff or painful, make the stretch gentler.

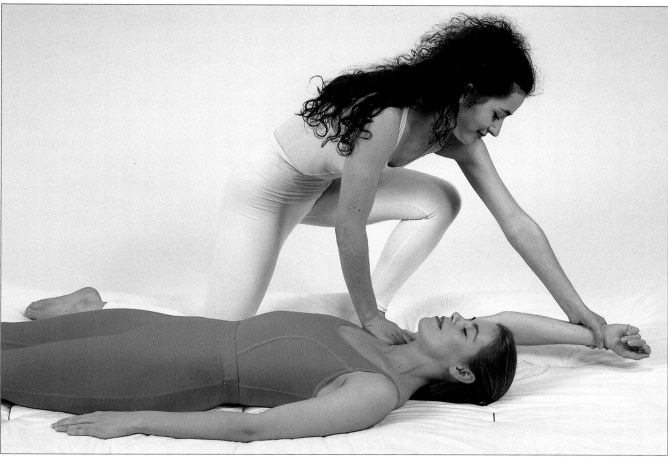

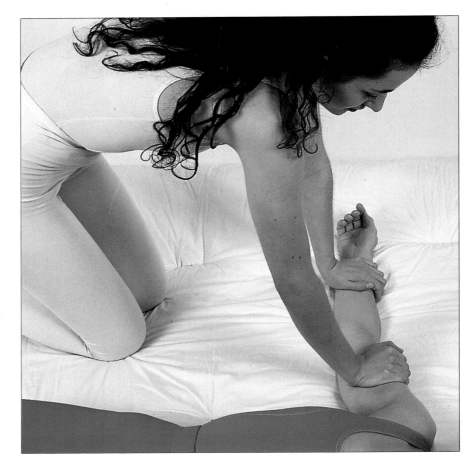

2 Switch to a kneeling position alongside your partner's waist. Lay the arm straight out perpendicular to the body, with the palm facing up. Place your far hand on the wrist, and apply palm pressure with your other hand (*right*), using the heel of your palm to press down, on the out-breath. Work from just below the shoulder down to the wrist. Do not apply pressure at the elbow. Repeat this two more times.

3 Pick up your partner's arm and, supporting their hand in yours, apply thumb pressure along three lines on the top surface of the upper arm (*right*), working from the top of the arm down to the elbow. These points can be found along the middle line of the muscle and to either side of the main muscle, along the edge of the bone. The points are shown at the bottom of the opposite page.

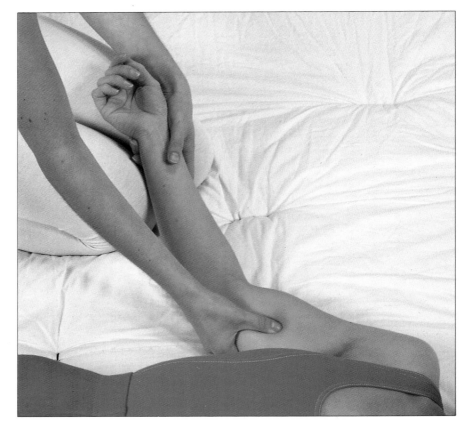

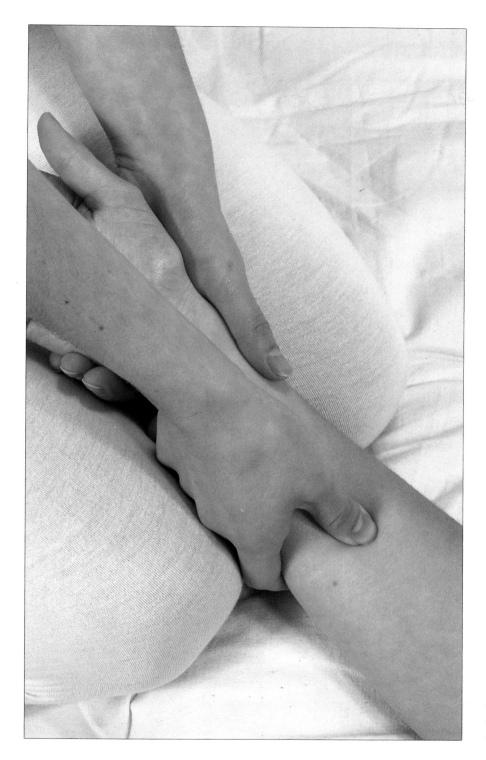

4 Continue this thumb pressure point work into the elbow and down to the wrist (*left*), as far as the creases at the base of the palm. Follow the same three lines worked on in the previous step above the elbow; the middle line falls along the centre of the muscles in the forearm, while the other two channels lie between these muscles and the inner bone edge on either side. Pay special attention to points that feel tender or seem blocked.

Inner arm pressure points
The lines of treatment used in steps 3 and 4 occur in three lines (*left*). As usual, press at intervals of a thumb's width.
Benefits: treatment of these points is particularly helpful to the heart and circulatory system, and to the lungs and respiratory system.

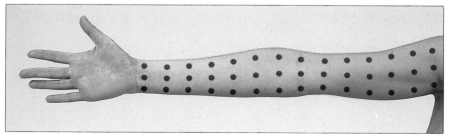

5 Now turn your partner's hand over, with the palm facing downwards, and bring the arm in closer to the body, so that it is almost parallel. Rotate your own body towards theirs to face this arm. With one hand on the wrist, begin to apply palm pressure from the wrist up towards the top of the arm with the other hand (*below*). Avoid direct pressure on the elbow as you palm up the arm. Notice that you are now working in the opposite direction from the previous steps on the arm. This is because the energy flows in the opposite direction in the meridians on the outside of the arm.

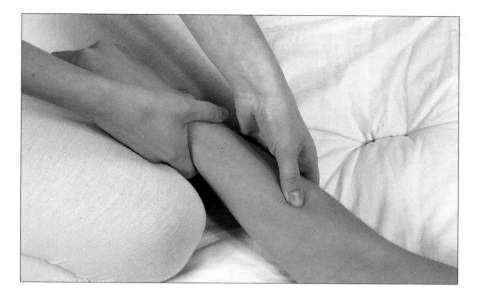

6 Support the arm by holding the hand, and apply thumb pressure over the outer surface of the lower arm, from the wrist up into the elbow (*left*). Remember not to apply pressure directly on the elbow. Follow three lines of pressure point work, shown at the bottom of this page. The middle line runs along the centre line of the muscle, midway between the two bones on either side, and the other two channels lie between the edges of this muscle mass and the two bones.

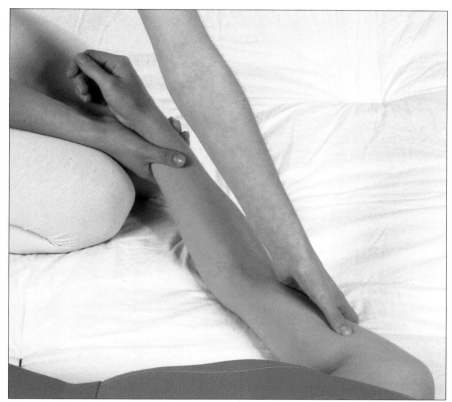

7 Continue thumb pressure along the outer surface of the upper arm, from the elbow to the shoulder (*left*). The middle line here runs centrally along the bone that you can feel in the upper arm, while the other two channels lie between this and the muscle tissue on either side. Finding these takes some practice. If you have difficulty locating the lines of pressures, ask your partner to tell you when they recognize the characteristic 'pressure-point sensation'.

Then move to the other side of the body, go back to page 79 and repeat steps 1–7 on your partner's other arm.

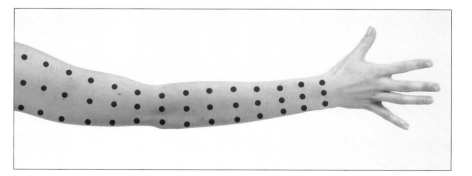

Outer arm pressure points
These three lines of treatment lie along the outer surface of the arm (*left*).
Benefits: particularly helpful for the large and small intestines, and the body metabolism in general.

9

THE CHEST AND NECK

The chest and neck can conveniently be treated as one sequence, although each has its own distinctive qualities. The chest comprises the rib-cage and collar-bone, and the upper organs, the heart and lungs, protected within the ribs, so work on the chest helps respiration and circulation. Many people hold suppressed emotion in the upper chest, especially those who have a habit of shallow breathing, Shiatsu can help to release such emotions. Sadness or grief is closely associated with the lungs and upper chest, and treatment can occasionally evoke tears. If this happens, assure your partner that it is perfectly all right.

The neck is not a self-contained entity; rather, it is the continuation of the spine into the skull. Nevertheless, it has its own particular significance and potential to reveal problems. It forms the bridge between the mind and body, between thoughts and emotions; so when there is lack of integration in these spheres, it often manifests in the neck. In fact, almost any kind of stress can appear here first; it is for good reason that we describe someone who causes us problems as 'a pain in the neck'. It is indeed a 'bottle-neck' through which blood and other vital fluids, nerve messages and Ki should flow freely; all too often blockages occur, resulting in stiffness, aches, pains or more serious neck problems. Excessive heat that you may feel in your partner's neck and tops of the shoulders is one indication of such blockage. Treatment of the neck helps free up this internal 'traffic'. In fact, the neck can serve as an early-warning system that indicates something going wrong, before it affects other parts of the body more profoundly.

The neck also serves to carry the weight of the head; if the rest of the body does not support it properly due to bad postural habits, then the neck is often affected first. In the oriental concept of correspondences between opposite parts, the neck is also considered to have a particularly close relationship with the lower back, sacrum, pelvis and also legs.

So discomfort in the neck nearly always indicates problems elsewhere in the body. Nevertheless, neck Shiatsu can contribute significantly, and usually provides a degree of instant relief. Serious neck problems should be referred to a chiropractor or osteopath.

About this sequence
The sequence here consists of loosening and opening stretches and then pressure-point work for first the chest and then the neck, leading directly on to the last lesson, treatment of the head and face. Some common problems that benefit from neck treatment include headaches, nervous tension, shoulder pain, low back pain, insomnia and hypertension.

POINTS TO REMEMBER
- *use your body weight, not muscular effort*
- *keep your own body relaxed*
- *focus attention and breathe in your abdomen*
- *keep your working arm straight but not locked*
- *lean into each movement on the out-breath, and hold the position*
- *work at right angles to the body surface*
- *cultivate a calm feeling and regular rhythm*

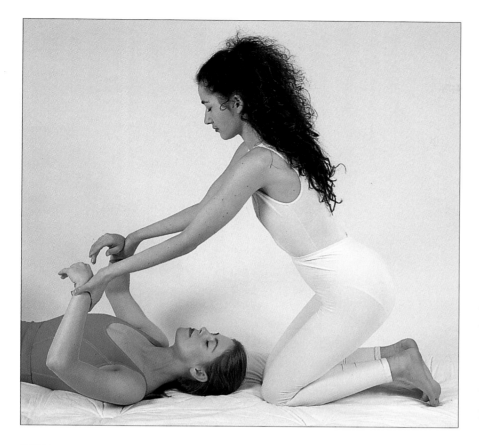

1 Kneel a little way above your partner's head. Lean over and pick up the hands (*left*). Ask your partner to relax and let go, and then to take an in-breath. As they do so, breathe in yourself, then sit back on your heels, taking up the tension in your partner's arms.

On an out-breath, lean backwards (*below*), allowing your arms to straighten, and use your body weight to produce a stretch in the shoulders and upper chest. Release on an in-breath and repeat twice more.

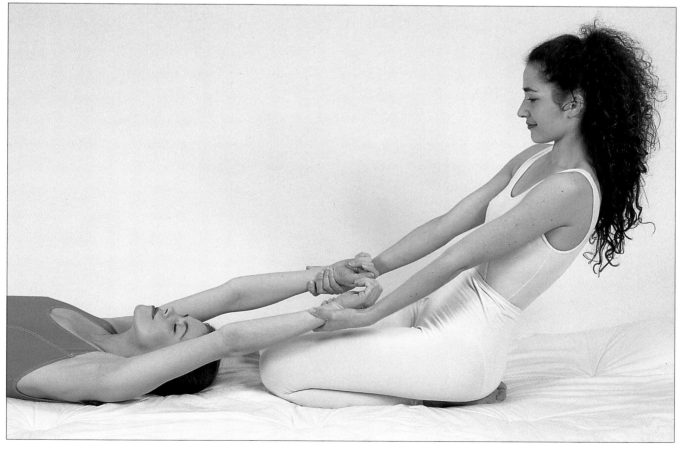

2 Come up off your heels and
place your hands on the top
surface of your partner's shoulders
with the heels of your hands
towards each other. Breathe in, and
lean downwards on an out-breath
(*right*), using your body weight.
Repeat twice more. Encourage your
partner to let go if you feel that
tension is being held in the
shoulders, and lean in more
strongly if you do not feel the
shoulders going down on to the
mattress. This can be a strong
stretch, which people usually find
pleasant. It also serves to make
your partner aware of the tension
they are holding in their shoulders,
and should encourage them to
relax further and let go.

3 Sit back on to your heels again,
and exert palm pressure over
the upper chest area, below the
collar-bone (*below*), from the
centre outwards and down on to
the lower ribs, with both hands at
once. Be careful to avoid applying
any pressure directly to breast
tissue while treating women.

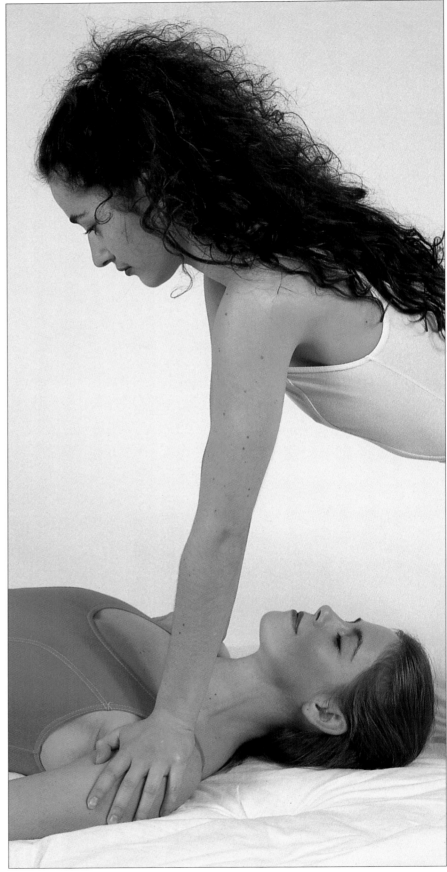

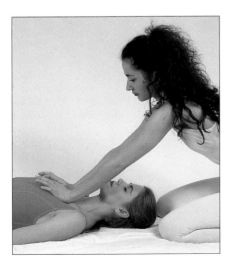

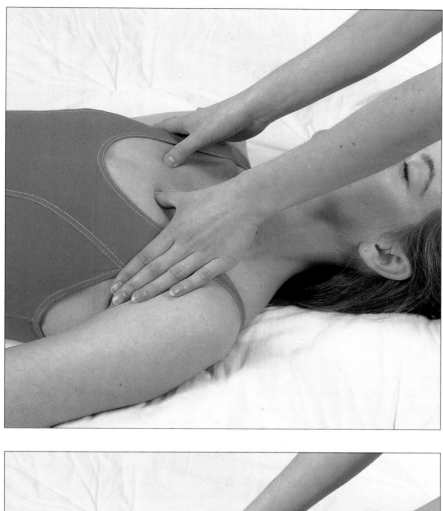

4 Now begin to apply thumb pressure to the chest (*left*). Work with both thumbs at once, which can make finding the points easier because of their symmetrical arrangement. Start just below the collar-bone. Find the line of points that are shown at the bottom of this page; each point is at the inner end of the hollow channel that runs between each rib. In the upper chest, these points are near the centre, just on either side of the sternum or breast-bone; further down the chest they diverge towards the sides. Again do not apply pressure to breast tissue in women.

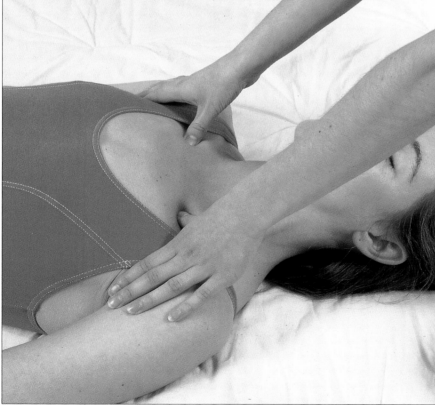

5 Starting again at the middle, on either side of the sternum, apply thumb pressure along the underside of the collar-bone (*left*), working out on to the front of the shoulders. Work again with both thumbs at once.

Chest pressure points
Lines of treatment for steps 4 and 5 are shown below.
Benefits: helps the lungs and breathing, and promotes release of chest tension and suppressed emotion; also helpful for asthma and lactation.

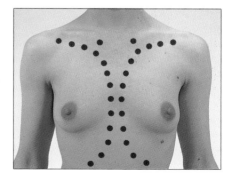

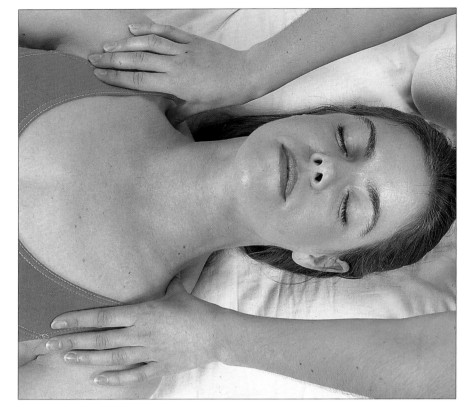

6 Apply thumb pressure along the tops of the shoulder muscles (*right*). You can work with both thumbs at once, or with one, keeping the other hand on the opposite shoulder. This technique is useful for shoulders that were still tense after the shoulder treatment in lesson 1, because the muscles are usually more relaxed in this position and at this stage in the treatment.

Shoulder pressure points
Treatment points appear below. *Benefits: helpful for shoulder and neck tension related headaches, numbness and 'frozen shoulder', and functioning of the intestines.*

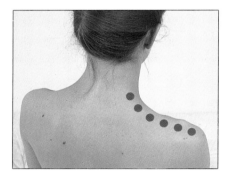

7 Place your hands under your partner's neck, asking them to allow the weight of the head to fall into your hands. Slowly draw the hands towards you in a rhythmic manner, one at time, keeping the head just off the mattress. The weight of the head provides the pressure required. Continue for a few moments, then rest your partner's head gently on the mattress.

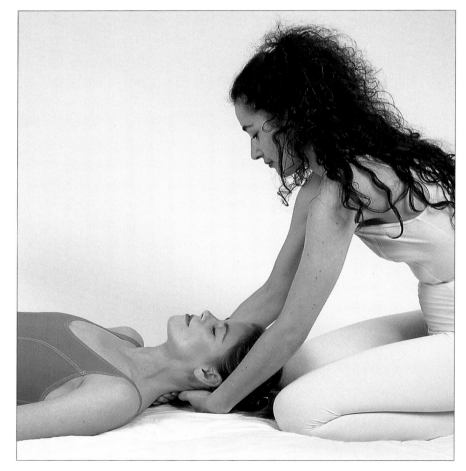

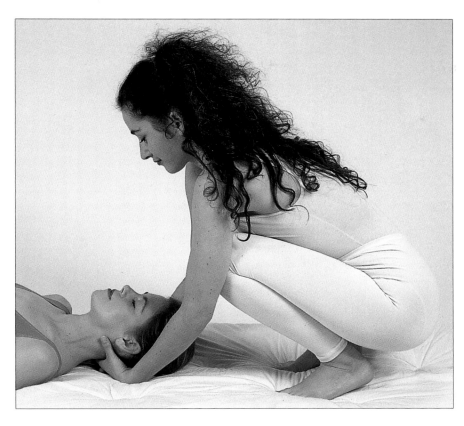

8 Now come up on to your feet, so that you are crouching just behind your partner's head. Place your hands under the neck again, but this time interlink your fingers just under the skull, with your thumbs catching the ledge just below the ears (*left*). Ask your partner to breathe in, and breathe in at the same time yourself.

On the out-breath for you both, let your body tilt back and your arms straighten, to give a strong stretch to the neck (*below*). Hold this for a full out-breath, then tilt forward again, and repeat twice more. You will know the stretch is complete when you see movement down to the feet. This stretch provides a valuable release for tension in the neck and shoulders, as well as in the upper back. It also helps open up the space between all the vertebrae.

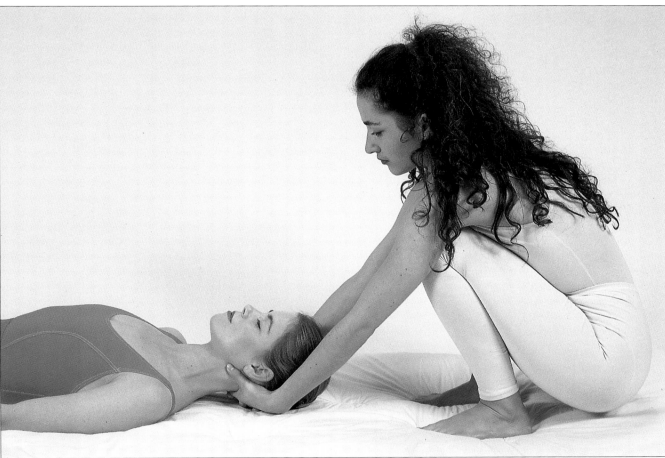

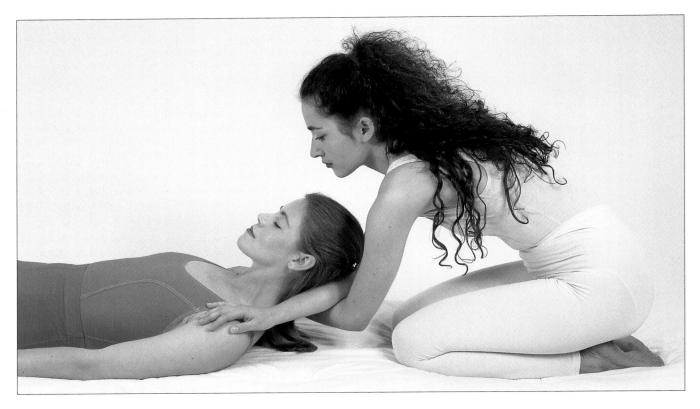

9 Revert to the kneeling position, cross your arms under your partner's head, place your right palm on your partner's left shoulder and your left palm on the right shoulder (*above*). Ask your partner to relax their neck and take an in-breath; take the weight of the head in the crook of your elbows. On the out-breath, raise your own body up from sitting (*right*), keeping your back straight, in order to bring a forward stretch into your partner's neck. Lower a little on the in-breath by sitting slightly, and repeat twice. You will probably find that the head goes a little further each time, but do not force it; just go to a comfortable stretch.

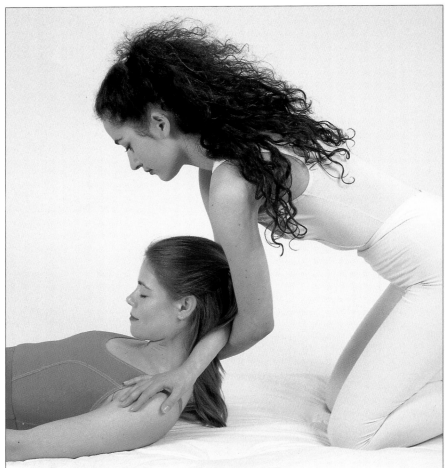

CAUTION

Do not perform this stretch if the neck is weak or injured, or if the receiver is suffering severe muscular pain in the neck.

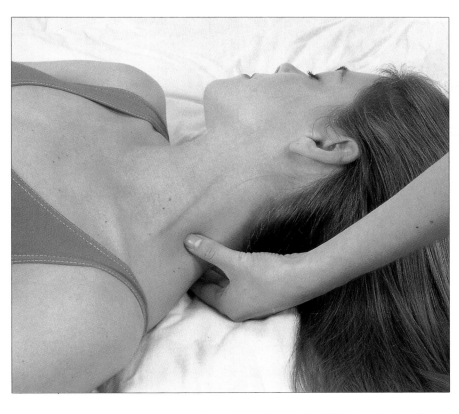

10 Sit back on your heels again, and turn your partner's head to the right; you can rest it either on the mattress or on your right hand. With your left hand, apply thumb pressure firmly along the line of the major muscle in the neck (*left*), from the junction with the shoulder up to the underside of the skull. If you find that this is very tense, you can prepare it with some kneading beforehand. The line of treatment is shown below. Repeat the pressures three times.

Neck and skull pressure points
Treat these points at intervals of one thumb width (*below*).
Benefits: helpful for insomnia, lateral headaches, neck tension, tinnitus, hangover and general stress. Also benefits the bladder, liver and gall bladder.

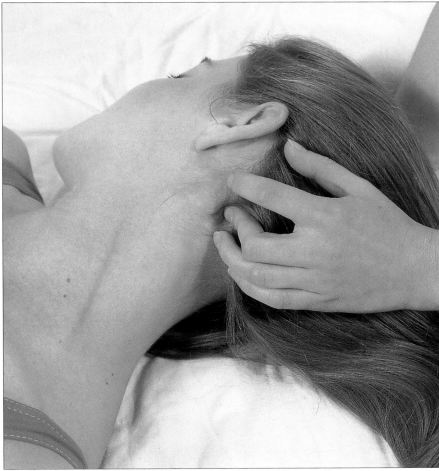

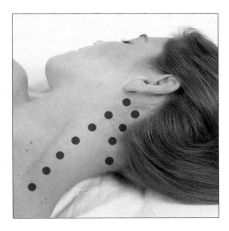

11 With the tips of your index and middle fingers, apply pressure along the base of the skull (*left*). Press right in under the ledge formed by the cranium. If some places seem blocked by muscular tension, apply circular massage with your fingers and then press in more strongly. This can take some time and may be painful if your partner is highly stressed, but will bring great relief.

Turn the head to the left, and repeat steps 10 and 11.

10

THE FACE

The face is a good place to finish a Shiatsu treatment; the lighter work is very pleasant after the strong stretches and deep point work on the rest of the body, some of which will inevitably have been uncomfortable.

The head contains the central focus for the nervous system, as well as the main sensory apparatus – the eyes, ears and nose – plus the entry points for food and air. We are very preoccupied with appearance in the West, so there are many related issues that Shiatsu work on the face helps to treat.

The preoccupation with the face and its appearance is not entirely misplaced. As all holistic therapies now recognize, and oriental medicine has long realized: the part reflects the whole, and the outside reflects the inside.

So the face reflects what is going on not only emotionally, but also physically, and in every other aspect of our being. Facial diagnosis is a science in itself, used by many Shiatsu practitioners (*see page 134*). Pay attention to the face while treating the rest of the body, to get an idea of the effects of your work.

About this sequence

The sequence here is a systematic procedure for treatment of points all over the face and on to the head. Go over everything three times. The points are treated symmetrically with both hands at once, unless otherwise stated. Points on the face relate to many different organs and parts of the body, so a comprehensive treatment of the face will benefit the whole system.

1 Kneeling behind your partner's head, as you did for work on the chest and neck, apply pressure with the two middle fingers along the lower edge of the cheek-bone (*right*). Start just in front of the lower part of ear and follow the ledge of bone in towards the nose. Press in under the bone. The line of treatment is shown at the bottom of the opposite page.

Make sure that your fingernails are cut short and have no sharp edges when carrying out this treatment. In the treatment of the face, you will no longer be leaning in with the whole body weight or keeping the arms straight. Because of the close work, it is necessary instead to use muscular effort in the arms, hands and fingers.

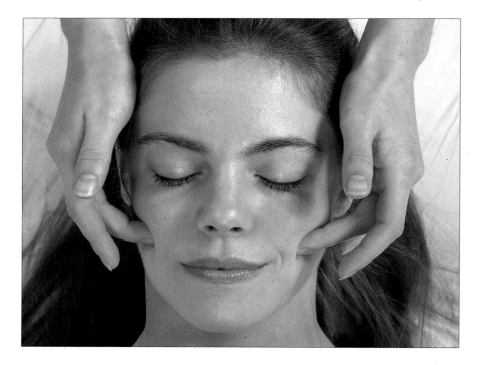

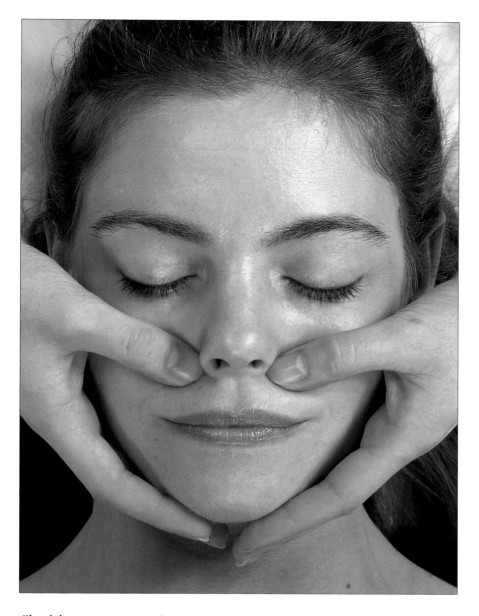

2 Apply pressure with the thumbs on the two points that lie in the hollows near the lower corners of the nostrils (*left*). Ask your partner to breathe in and take a breath yourself at the same time. As you breathe out together, press in strongly and repeat twice more, on each out-breath. The fingers can lie under the chin to keep the hands steady while you are locating the points.

Cheek-bone pressure points
The lines of treatment are around the base of the cheek-bone (*right*). Press at intervals of approximately a thumb's width. *Benefits: these points are especially helpful for sinus congestion, but also relate to the large intestine and stomach.*

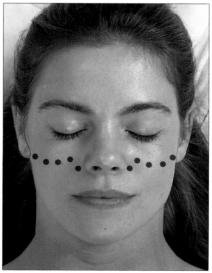

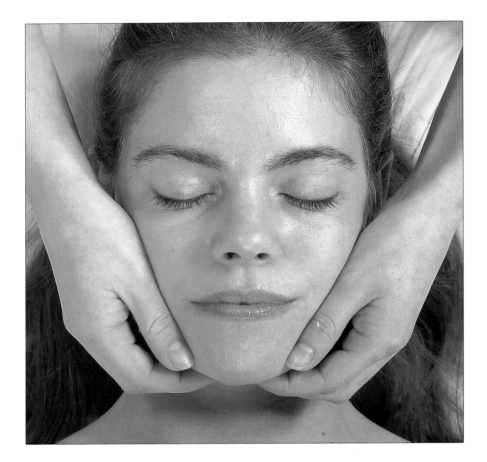

3 Bring your hands down to the chin. With the thumbs on the front of the chin, press in under the jaw-bone with the tips of the first and second fingers (*right*). Proceed from the centre outwards, along the underside of the jaw, at intervals of a thumb's width, until you reach the ear.

4 Turn the head to one side. With the index finger of one hand, press into the point which lies in the hollow underneath the earlobe (*right*). This point is very tender in some people, so be aware of your partner's reaction. Turn the head the other way and repeat.

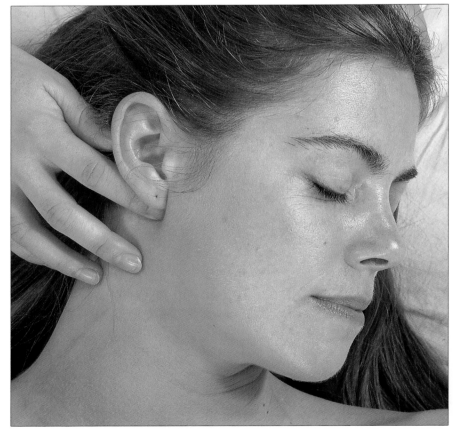

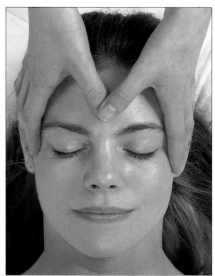

5 With one thumb on top of the other at the centre of the forehead, and anchoring your fingers around the sides of the head (*right*), apply pressure in a line, starting between the eyebrows and continuing onto the top of the head.

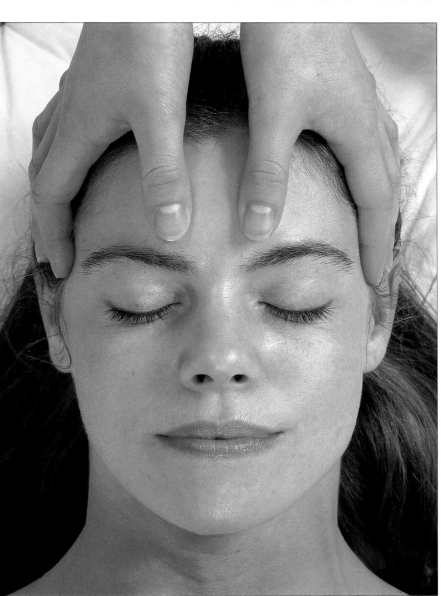

6 Again, anchoring your fingers around the sides of your partner's head, position your thumbs at the inner ends of the eyebrows. Apply thumb pressure in two lines straight up from the eyebrows (*left*), continuing with your thumbs at this spacing, up on to the top of the head.

Forehead pressure points
Work the lines of treatment for steps 5 and 6 (*below*) at intervals of one thumb width.
Benefits: helpful to the bladder; helps release headache and tension in the front of the head, as well as calming the mind.

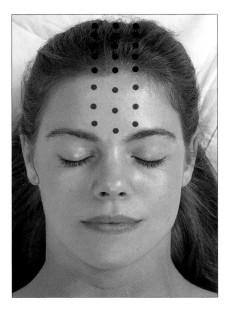

95

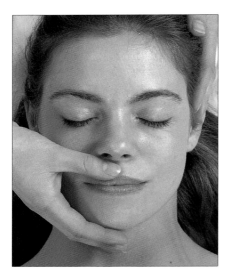

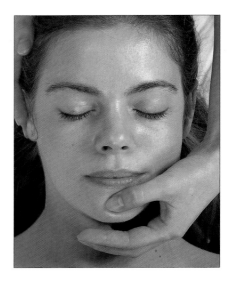

7 Apply thumb pressure to the point just below the centre of the nose (*left*), and to the point below the centre of the mouth (*right*), in the hollow at the roots of the teeth. Remember to apply all the pressures three times on the out-breaths. Support the head with your passive hand.

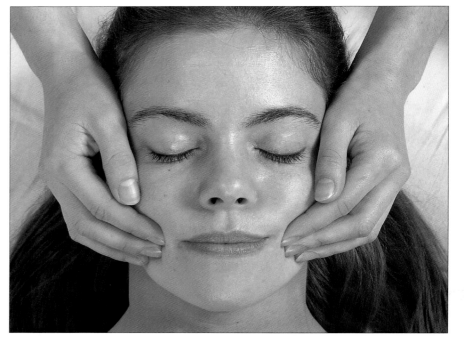

8 Steadying your hands against your partner's head, with the tips of the first and second fingers, apply pressure all around the mouth (*right*). Search for the points at the roots of the teeth about 2–3 centimetres (1 inch) out from the lips.

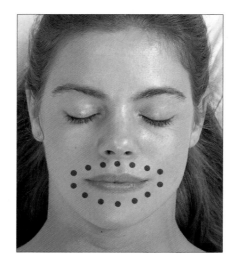

Mouth pressure points
Work around the line of treatment for step 8 (*left*) at intervals of approximately one thumb width, as usual.
Benefits: particularly helpful to the stomach and large intestine, also stimulate salivation, appetite and digestion.

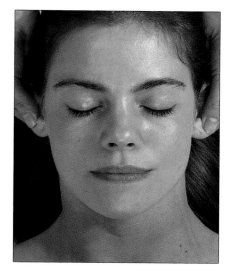

9 Treat the ears by squeezing (*left*), pulling and stretching, the whole way around and all over the outer ear. This can be done firmly and comprehensively, and feels surprisingly pleasant. The ear is another 'model' of the body, containing a large number of treatment points that cover the whole system.

10 Strongly pinch the eyebrows, from the inner to the outer edges (*below*). This can be very relaxing, especially for tired eyes; it also helps to relieve stress or tension. Make sure your fingernails are not too long for this, and be careful to avoid putting pressure on the eyelids. Repeat this three times in total.

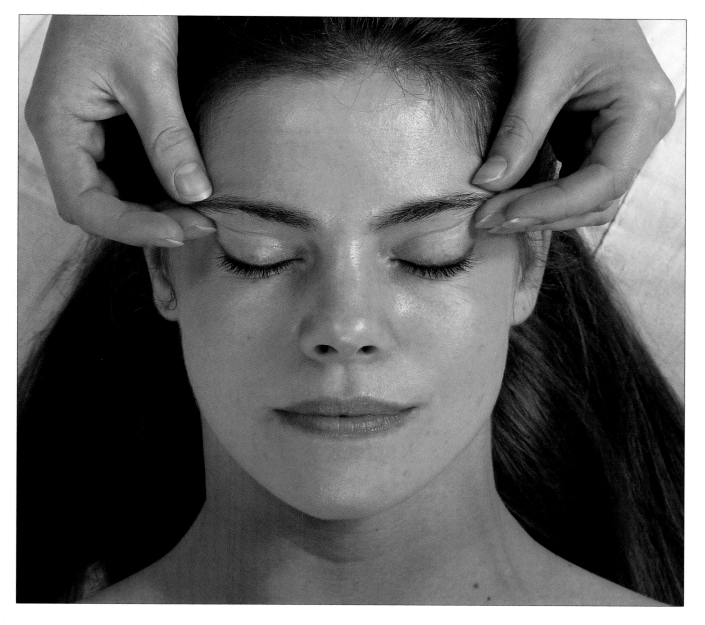

11 Massage the forehead by stroking across it, using the length of your thumbs laid down on the forehead (*right*). Start above the eyebrows at the inside end, and draw the thumbs out towards the temples. Repeat this several times, pressing strongly at first and finishing with lighter strokes.

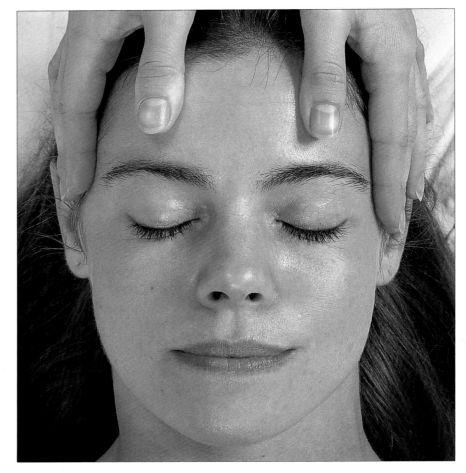

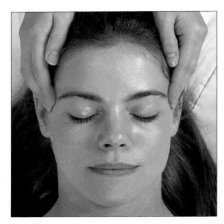

12 Massage the temples, with the tips of the first and second fingers (*above*), in a circular motion, pressing strongly at first and finishing with a very light action.

13 Finally, grasp tufts of your partner's hair (*right*), and tug them gently towards you. Start in the front, at the centre of the forehead, and work around the hairline as far as you can, towards the back of the head. Then work around again in concentric circles, a little further in each time, so that you are treating the whole scalp, finishing at the crown – the point where a line drawn up from the ears would intersect with a line from the nose. This gives a pleasant conclusion to the treatment of the head, and draws your partner's energy upwards. You can follow this with the finishing sequence shown on page 100.

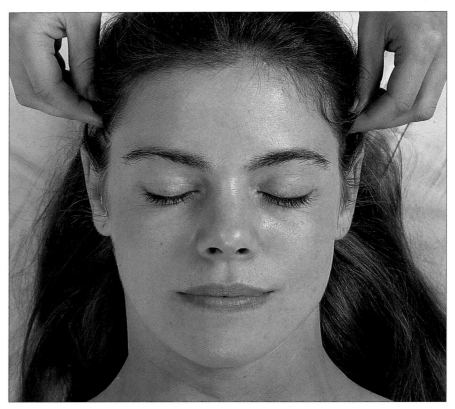

FINISHING A TREATMENT

To complete any Shiatsu sequence where your partner is lying down, use the two steps shown overleaf. Whatever type of Shiatsu you have given, there are a number of factors to consider upon finishing: some relating to your partner and some to yourself.

Caring for your partner

After any comprehensive treatment, let your partner relax for about five minutes, while you leave the room. The deep state of relaxation induced by Shiatsu can be healing in itself and the effects can go on working; people often report that they can feel areas being worked on after the pressure has been released. As peripheral circulation withdraws, the surface of the body cools dramatically, so make sure that your partner is warm enough; cover them with a blanket or duvet if necessary.

When you rejoin your partner it is a good idea to discuss the treatment. Ask them for feedback, so that you can both learn from the practice and understand the condition better for future treatments. Find out which parts of your work felt good to them and which, if any, were uncomfortable. Remember that not all the benefit is felt immediately, and that some points inevitably feel tender – especially the ones that most need treatment. If you can, check how they feel in a few days. If they had lasting aches and pains or a bruised feeling, then you were probably working too strongly.

As you practise more, you will also be able to give your partner feedback about your findings during the session – the state of Ki flow, general well-being or health of different parts of the body – particularly when you have studied Part Three.

The nervous system can remain in the same deeply relaxed state even after the body has resumed activity. Reflexes can be slow, so the receiver should take extra care, especially when driving or crossing roads. In fact, they will gain maximum benefit from a full treatment by taking it easy for the rest of the day. People who have been feeling very weak for some time, and then feel energized from Shiatsu, should take particular care not to squander this energy by immediately doing all the things they have been too exhausted to do. They need to continue at a slow pace for some time, in order to build up their resources.

Finally, point out to your partner that a 'reaction' can occasionally occur in the twenty-four hours after a Shiatsu treatment. This is the result of discharge of toxicity into the bloodstream, and release of Ki blockages (*see page 9*). It is a good idea for your partner to drink a glass of pure water after any Shiatsu to facilitate elimination of toxins.

Looking after yourself

Wash your hands immediately after giving Shiatsu; even if they are clean, rinse them in cold water, and shake until dry. This helps disperse any unhealthy energies you may have picked up. Many people eliminate toxins, both physically through the skin and also as energy discharge; you may find this tiring while you are new to Shiatsu. Do some exercises to help you renew your energies, such as visualizations, yoga stretches or meditation, and then rest if you need to. Self-shiatsu or energizing exercises can also help (*see pages 103–115*).

It is also important to clear the energies in the room – much as you may have done before beginning, with incense or candles – especially if you are going to start on another treatment, or if the room is about to revert to another purpose.

Right. *Sit alongside your partner and place one hand on the abdomen and one on the upper chest. These correspond to the major upper and lower internal energy centres: the Tan Den and the heart chakra. Hold this position for a few moments. Breathe calmly and naturally into your abdomen, and hold an image of peacefulness and healing for your partner's whole being. This brings a unifying and balancing effect to the overall Ki system, after your work on all the different body zones, organ systems and Ki channels.*

Below. *Finally, stand alongside your partner's feet, and sweep your hands several times over the whole body a few inches above the body's surface, starting at the feet and working up to the head. This draws energy up through the body's external energy field or aura, in preparation for rising shortly.*

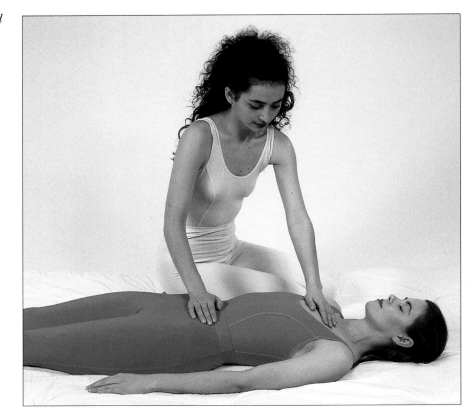

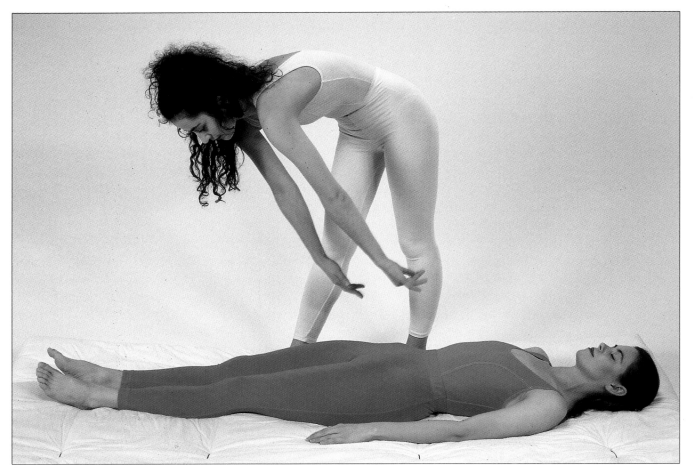

MINI TREATMENTS

It is not always possible, or necessary, to carry out the whole sequence; much can be achieved in shorter, more focused sessions. Furthermore, some people may wish to try a sample before committing to a full body treatment. At other times, lying on the floor may be inappropriate or impossible. If so, or if time is limited, a partial treatment can be used. You will also find that you have to adapt some techniques to individual circumstances, for instance to treat an elderly or injured person who cannot lie down in certain positions.

In fact, Shiatsu to certain parts of the body can still have a comprehensive effect on the whole system, for many parts contain treatment areas for the whole. So here are some options for shorter treatments.

Shoulders

A shoulder treatment is an ideal introduction to Shiatsu. It can be carried out anywhere that there is a chair or floor space to sit on, and can be very quick or relatively thorough. Treating the shoulders can bring impressive effects in a short time. If you choose to give a sitting-position Shiatsu, you can extend the shoulder treatment by working on the upper back and on the neck and head, adapting the techniques from the relevant lessons. A shoulder mini-treatment is particularly appropriate for any tension in the upper body or for headaches.

Back and shoulders

The back is a primary candidate for treatment when time is limited, containing as it does treatment points for all the major organs. It is also an area where many people experience problems. As well as following lesson 2, you could add an adapted shoulder massage by working from alongside the back, and shoulder point work by sitting above your partner's head while they are lying face-down.

Face, head, neck and shoulders

For someone suffering upper body tension or headache, who would like a more informal treatment, this is a good alternative. Lessons 9 and 10 cover these areas.

Back of body

Covering the whole of the back of the body gives your partner a more comprehensive sense of treatment than working only on the back. Do include the feet to complete this effect; you need not turn your partner over, just adapt the foot treatment to enable you to work on the top surface and toes. This sequence is useful if there is tension in the back of the body, and if your partner likes stronger work. It will take about 20–25 minutes.

Front of body

Treating the whole of the front of the body also benefits all major body systems, and may be more appropriate where there are frontal problems, for instance in the abdominal area. Start with the shoulders, and work down to the feet, including work on both hands and feet, and finishing with the face. Again, you will need to adapt your technique to treat the soles of the feet from this position.

Feet only

This is a popular and enjoyable treatment in itself, which many people find very sensuous. If you are just doing the feet, your partner might prefer to sit in a comfortable chair with their feet raised on a stool. The feet are also prime candidates for self-Shiatsu.

Hands only

The hands can be given Shiatsu in almost any situation; regular treatment is very helpful for arthritis. Again, self-treatment is easy, and more discrete, so can be used in more places. It is particularly useful for revitalization during the day.

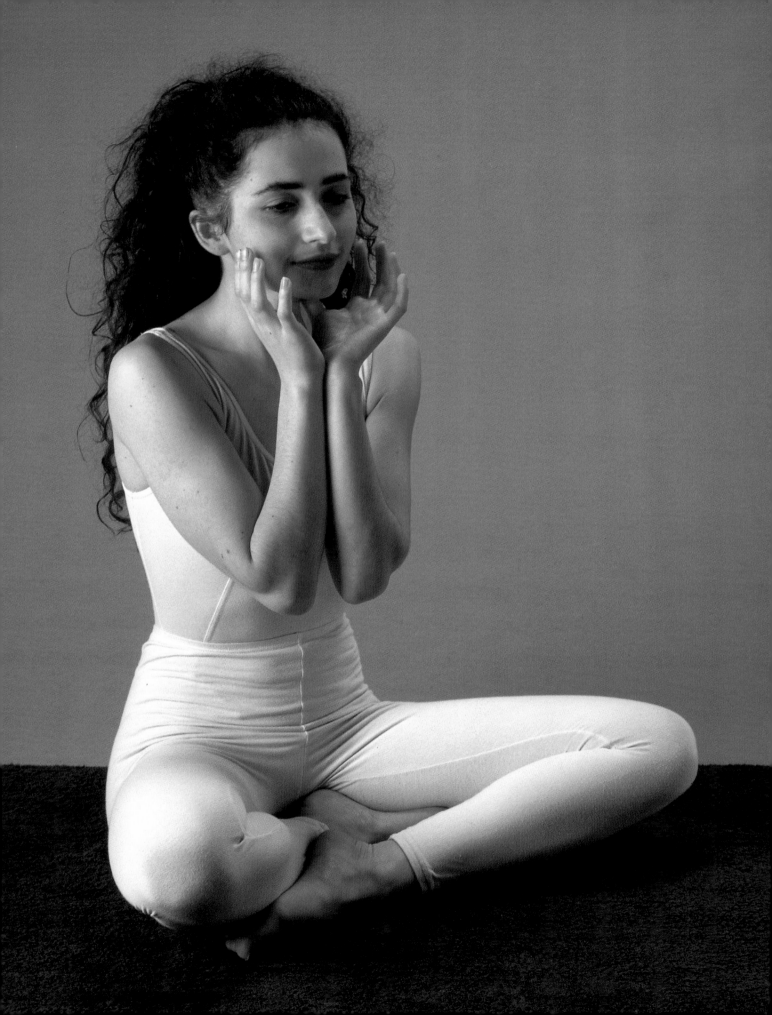

PART TWO

SELF-TREATMENT

One of the great advantages of Shiatsu is that you can use it for your own benefit as readily as you can to help other people. In fact, by treating yourself you will learn a great deal that will enhance your technique; you can experiment with locating pressure points more precisely, and you can discover what they feel like when treated, and how much pressure is appropriate for each one. Of course, when treating yourself you cannot reach all the points, especially those on the back, or apply the overall stretches or rotations in quite the same way. However, you can easily adapt the palming and thumbing techniques for the limbs and the front of the body. This means that you can carry out a comprehensive self-treatment that includes representative sections of all the major Ki channels, covering all the main body organs.

This part of the book does not repeat the whole sequence of techniques in Part One for self-treatment; rather it gives guidelines and examples of adaptation, together with some additional classical routines that have evolved specifically for one-person Shiatsu. The material is arranged in the order that best suits a complete self-treatment: a series of overall stretches to release tension, promote overall Ki flow and prepare for more specific work, first; a quick self-treatment sequence for the channels of the whole body, which can also serve as a framework for more detailed portions of self-treatment, next; and lastly, an example of detailed adaptation of a conventional Shiatsu routine for self-treatment, which also forms a useful finishing sequence, on the face and head. Naturally, any part of this overall plan can also be used on its own.

Left. *Adapting Shiatsu techniques for self-treatment is easy. This photograph shows how to modify pressure-point work for application around the jaw.*

SHIATSU STRETCHES

The six 'meridian' stretches that follow can form the start of a comprehensive self-treatment, or can be used as a set of exercises in their own right. Alternatively, you could use them as a preparation for giving Shiatsu, or even take your partner through them with you before starting a session. Whichever the application the key quality is that, together, they comprehensively stretch and stimulate all the major internal energy channels in turn; they help dissolve stagnation, remove blockages, promote flow through the body and help balance Ki levels between the different organ systems. The whole sequence takes about ten minutes to complete, depending on how long each stretch is held.

If you are very stiff or have just got up in the morning, it is advisable to loosen up before starting the stretches. It is important to take the posture only to the point where you feel a comfortable stretch.

1a There is a basic pattern to each of these stretches: first you go into a preliminary position and draw an in-breath; then you move into the stretch position on an out-breath; maintain the stretch for the out-breath, and release on the next in-breath. Then go into the stretch again on another out-breath and hold it for a number of in- and out-breaths, coming out of the stretch position on a final in-breath. In the stretch position, the body as a whole should be relaxed and the breathing natural, regular and continuous; the period of stretching lasts until you can feel energy flowing along the lines of stretch related to that particular exercise. This usually takes about thirty seconds, but can take up to several minutes. On the second stretch, you will usually be able to go a little further.

This stretch particularly stimulates the lungs and large intestine. It has several stages; to prepare for it, stand with your fingers interlinked behind your back (*right*), and breathe in.

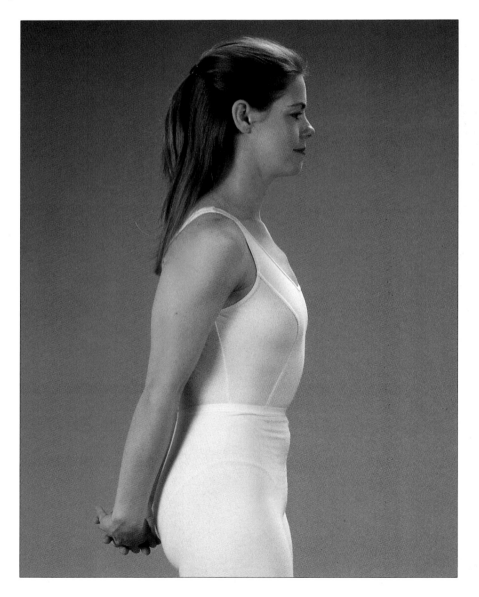

1b On the out-breath, bend forward from the waist (*below*), pushing your arms away from your body. On an in-breath, soften the stretch; and on the next out-breath stretch again and hold the stretch, breathing deeply and naturally. Release and return to an upright position on an in-breath. Then repeat the procedure, this time bending backwards from the waist (*left*), again stretching the arms away from the body. Finally, interlink your fingers again, but this time so that the thumb that was previously on top is now underneath, with each finger moving accordingly.

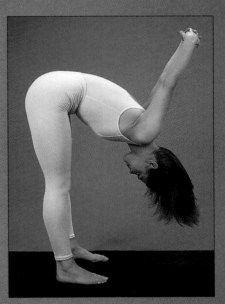

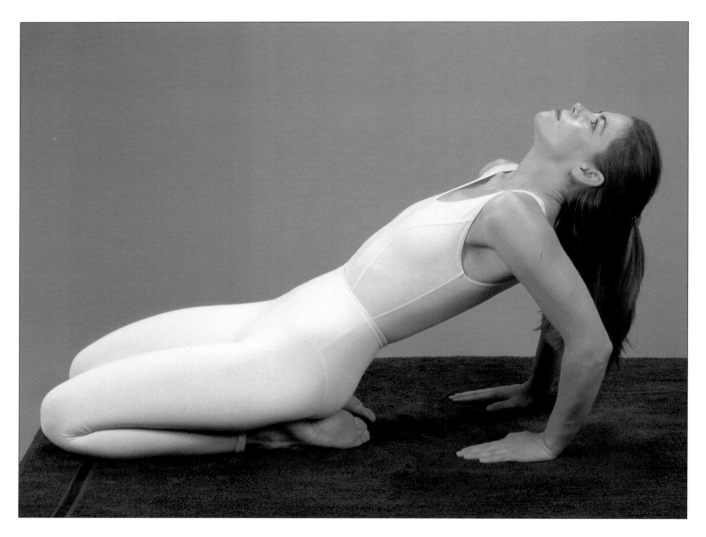

2a This stretch can be varied to suit your degree of flexibility. As it stimulates the stomach, spleen and pancreas, it is not appropriate soon after eating.

Kneel and lean backwards, placing your hands on the floor behind (*above*). Then either 'breathe and stretch' in this position, or lean back further, if you can, to a more advanced position (*middle, bottom right and top opposite*), and do so there. The sequence is as follows: breathe in; on an out-breath, lower the body a little, bringing a stretch into the front of the body; on an in-breath, soften the stretch; and on the next out-breath stretch again and hold, breathing naturally. Release and come out of the position by rolling to one side (*middle opposite*) on an in-breath.

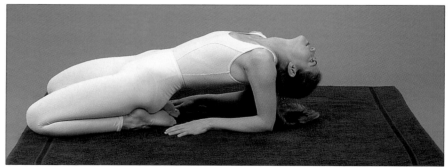

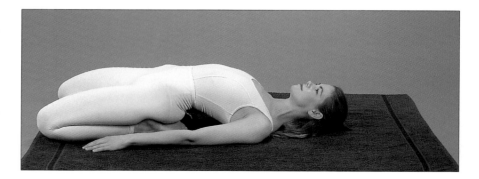

106

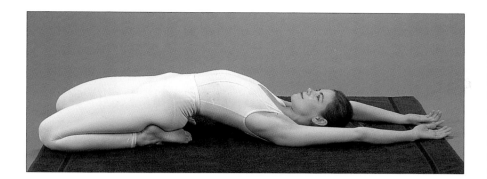

2b The most strenuous version of this stretch is to take the back down flat on the floor, by taking the feet wider apart, and to bring the arms over the head (*left*). Only do this if you have done similar postures in yoga, or are confident that you are supple enough. This stretch is mainly felt along the front of the body, particularly the legs.

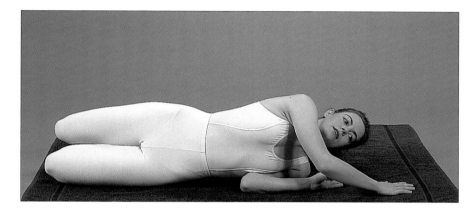

2c Especially if you have gone as far as the version shown in 2b, it is important to come out of the position by rolling over sideways (*left*) and coming up on to all fours as you breathe in. If you were to come up forwards, it would put great strain on the back and abdomen.

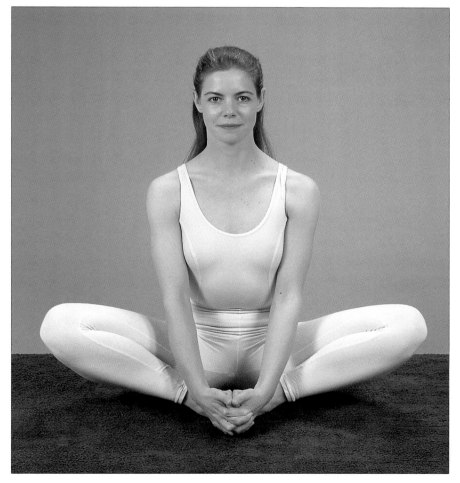

3a The third stretch benefits the heart and the small intestine. Start by sitting up straight with the feet drawn up to the groin and the soles together (*left*). Clasp your hands around the feet.

3b For the stretch position, lean forward (*below*), on an out-breath, keeping your elbows in front of your legs. Hold, and on the in-breath soften the stretch; resume the stretch on the next out-breath and maintain it breathing naturally for a few moments. If you have back problems, bend from the waist, keeping the upper back straight. You should feel the stretch in the inner arms.

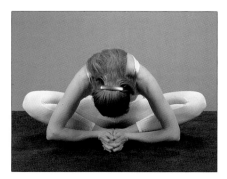

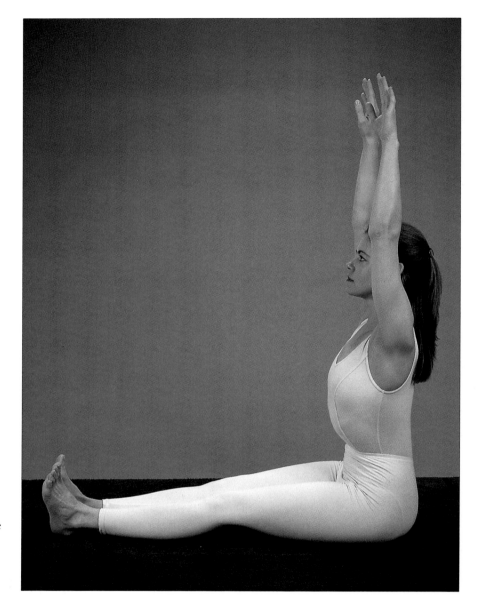

4a This stretch relates to the kidneys and bladder. Prepare for the stretch by sitting with your legs straight out in front and reaching, with your arms, up over your head (*right*). Breathe in.

4b Stretch on the out-breath by reaching forward, placing your hands on your lower legs, on your ankles, or over the tops of your feet (*right*) – whichever is a comfortable stretch. You will feel the stretch over the outside of the body: down the back and in the backs of the legs. Soften the stretch on the next in-breath, then resume the stretch as you breathe out continuing to breath in a relaxed way as you hold the stretch for a short time.

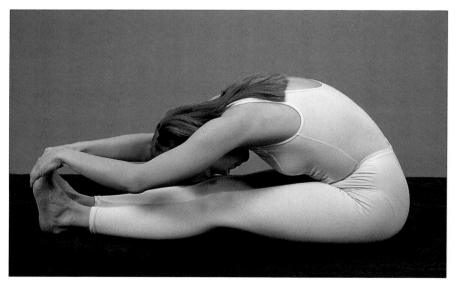

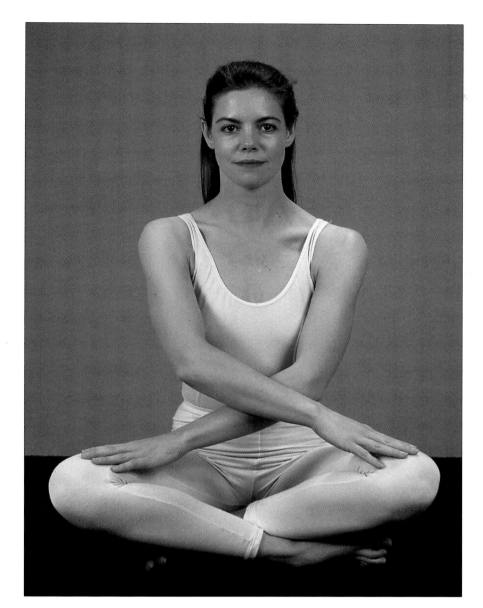

5a This stretch is related to the Heart Governor and Triple Heater (*see page 126*) and has two stages. It helps to regulate circulation, metabolism and heat in the body. Start by sitting with the legs crossed, or with the soles of the feet together if this is more comfortable. Cross the arms, and place one hand over each knee (*left*). Breathe in.

5b To create the stretch, bend forward on the out-breath, holding on to your knees, dropping your head downwards, and letting your knees travel towards the floor (*below*). You should feel this stretch in the front and back surfaces of the arms. As usual, soften the stretch, then stretch again for a little longer. For the second stage, sit upright again, re-cross the legs and arms so that the other one is on top, and repeat the stretching and breathing procedure.

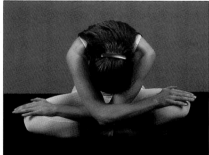

6 The final stretch benefits the liver and the gall bladder. Sit with legs spread widely, and fold your right leg in towards the groin. Lean over to the left, facing forward, and place your hand on your leg, palm-up (*left*). For the stretch, bring the right arm over your head. You can get a stronger stretch by keeping both legs spread apart. Repeat the whole sequence for the other side by folding in your left leg and leaning over to the right. This completes the stretches.

Now lie on your back for a few minutes, relax and observe energy sensations in the body.

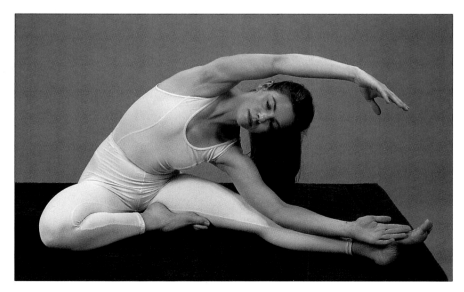

109

SELF-SHIATSU

This section presents a short routine for self-treatment, which can also form a basic framework for more detailed treatment, to which you can add further work adapted from the Shiatsu sequence in Part One. The basic procedure is taken from the classical oriental art of self-development and Ki enhancement known as 'Do-In', which is traditionally used as a warm-up in martial arts and Shiatsu classes. The Ki channels are treated all over the body, mainly with pounding techniques, to enhance flow of energy and tone up the muscles. This sequence can also be used as a gentle exercise programme in its own right, or as a loosening-up preparation for any other exercise regime, such as yoga or aerobics.

Examples of Shiatsu technique that can be readily adapted for self-treatment and worked into the Do-In routine follow.

The face and head
Detailed point work is covered on pages 116–119. It is particularly easy to adapt Shiatsu for the face and head, and it is very soothing.

The shoulders
You can easily do self-massage and pressure-point work on yourself, by working on each shoulder with the opposite hand; resting the elbow in your palm as you do so. This position is shown, for Do-In, in step 3 on page 112. Pressure can usually be applied more easily with the fingertips than with the thumbs.

The legs
Sitting on the floor is a good position for self-treatment of the legs. Sit on the right buttock, and bend both legs towards the left, with one slightly in front of the other; this position allows you to palm and then do point work to the inside and back of the right leg, and to the outside and front of the left leg. Then turn the legs the other way to complete the treatment.

In this position, you can lean in with the upper body weight, focusing in the abdomen, having an active and a passive hand and keeping the working arm straight.

The arms
Access to the arms is straightforward, but since you cannot lay the treated arm on the floor, instead you can hold it against the body as a support. You can use thumb pressure on the upper and outer surfaces, and fingertip pressure on the less accessible areas.

The hands and feet
Treatment of your own hands and feet is much the same as treating someone else's. Sit with one leg straight out in front and the ankle of the other leg across the thigh; this gives easy access to the sole of the foot. To treat the top of that foot place it flat on the floor, drawing it close enough to reach easily.

Guidelines for the Do-In sequence
Keep your whole body relaxed during this sequence, particularly the part you are working on, and proceed in a lively manner. Breathe naturally and continuously throughout. Pound with a lightly-clenched fist, making sure the wrist is floppy; you can work quite vigorously in this way, without causing pain or bruising.

The direction of work enhances the overall pattern of Ki flow in the body – upwards on the front and the inner surfaces of the limbs, and downwards on the back and outer limb surfaces. The sequence starts with the head, then shoulders, proceeding to the arms, then back, buttocks and legs, to the abdomen and finally the chest. At this point you can go on to the detailed treatment of the face, which starts on page 116. At any point in the sequence, you can bring in the detailed palming and point work just described.

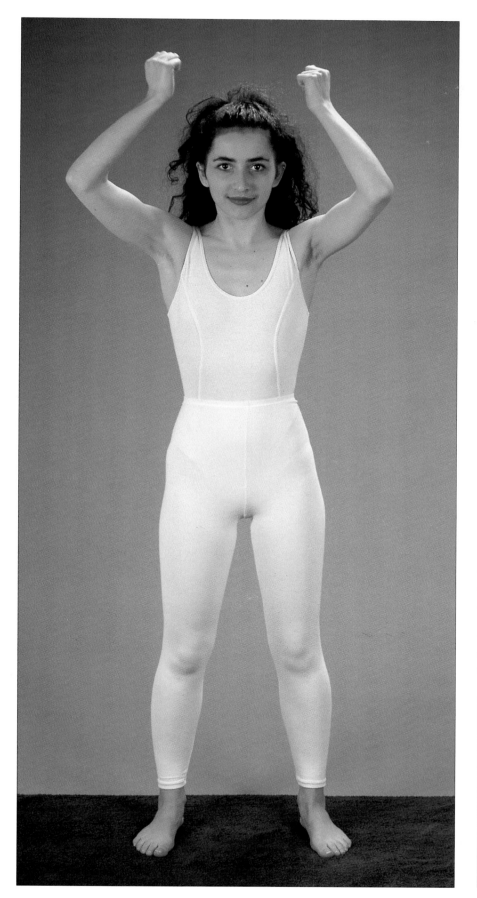

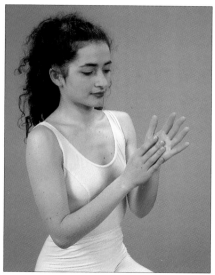

1 Rub your hands together vigorously, in front of you, for a few moments (*above*). You should cover the whole hand and the wrist as you do this, and continue until you feel energy in the hands (*see page 123*). Energizing the hands in this way will enhance the effect on Ki flow in the body.

2 Standing up with your feet slightly apart, pound over the head, using either the fists (*left*) always keeping the wrists floppy, or the flat of the hands (*below*) if the head feels more delicate. Start at the front in the middle and work backwards, first in two lines over the centre of the head, then further out towards the sides of the head, and so on until you have covered the whole surface. Remember to allow the breath to flow in a continuous, natural pattern.

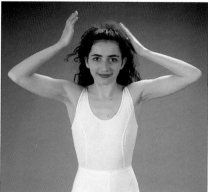

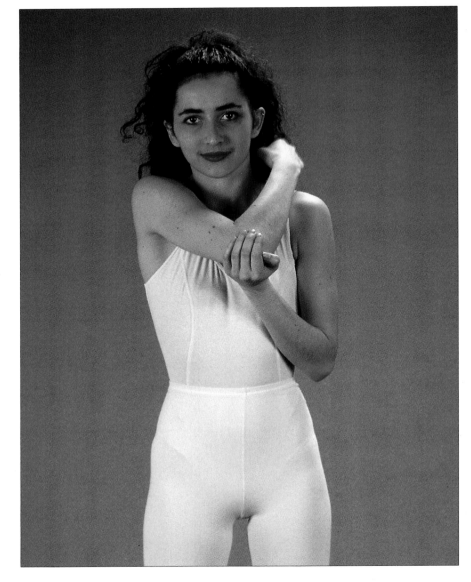

3 Support your right elbow with your left hand, tucking your left upper arm into your body (*right*), and pound vigorously on the muscles of the left shoulder with the right fist, remembering not to clench it too tightly and to keep the wrist floppy. Cover the whole area of the shoulder and up into the base of the neck. Continue pounding for about thirty seconds, or until the area feels loosened. Then swap arms and pound the right shoulder with the left fist, breathing all the time in a relaxed and continuous manner.

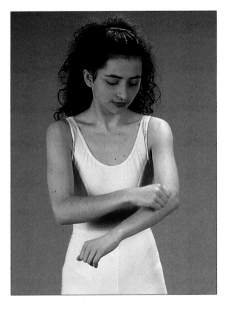

4 Holding your arm out in front of you with the palm facing downwards, pound along the upper surface of the arm (*left*), starting at the wrist and working up to the shoulder. Repeat at least three times. Then turn the arm over, so that the palm faces upwards, and pound along the inner surface of the arm (*right*), this time from the armpit down to the wrist. Again, repeat at least three times.

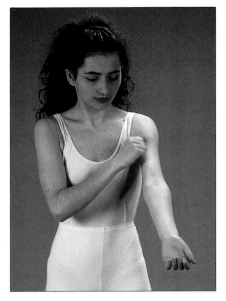

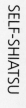

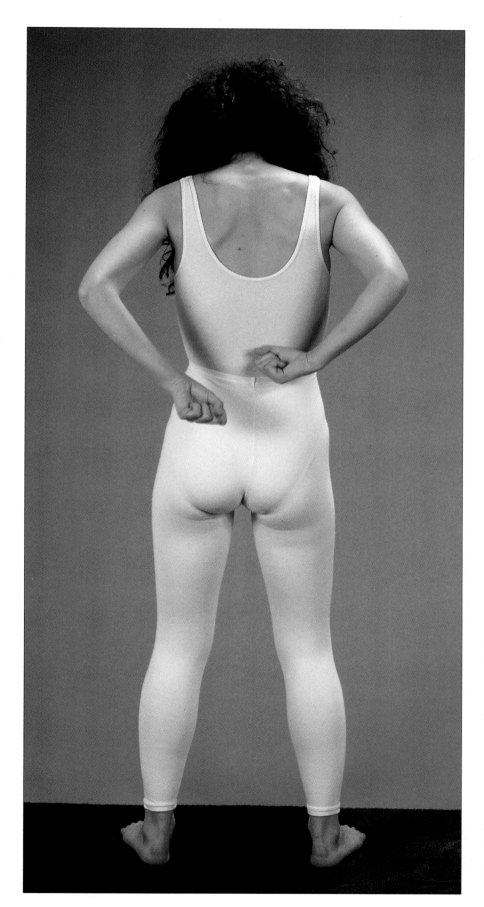

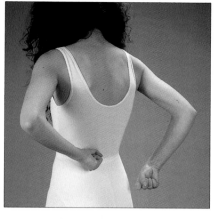

5 Pound down either side of the spine (*left*), from as high as you can reach behind your back, down on to the sacrum. Use the front of the fists – the thumb and curled forefinger (*above*). Alternate the fists in a continuous, rapid rhythm, remembering to keep the wrists floppy. Pound down the two sides three times. Doing this as a regular exercise, especially in the mornings, can help prevent straining the back during the day.

6 Pound very strongly all over the buttocks (*below*), again in a rapid, alternating rhythm, and again with the fronts of the fists. This exercise helps eliminate the stagnation of Ki which can build up in this area as a result of a sedentary lifestyle.

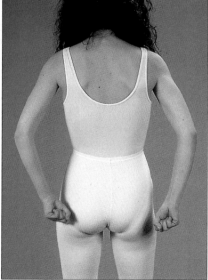

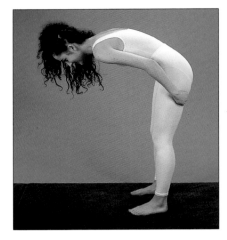

7 Bend forward, keeping the legs slightly bent so that the muscles are not tensed and the knees are not locked. In this position, pound all the way down the backs and outsides of the legs (*above*) from the buttocks to the ankles with the fronts of the fingers. Then pound up the fronts and insides of the legs (*right*) from the ankles to the thighs. Remember not to clench the fist and keep the wrist floppy whilst pounding. Repeat this procedure another two times.

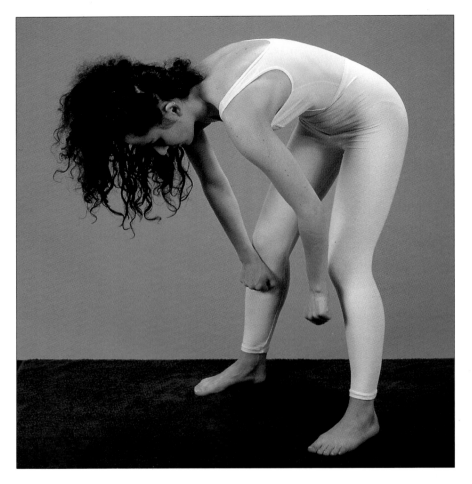

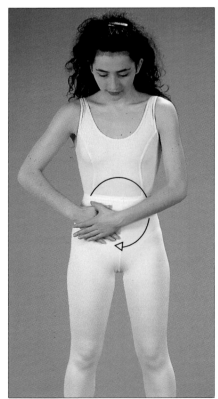

8 Massage the abdomen. Starting in the lower right region, between the pubic bone and the corner of the pelvis, place one hand on top of the other (*left*); press in strongly, and then move the hands round the abdominal cavity, in a clockwise circle centred on the navel. Do this at least three times. This exercise is not only helpful for the intestines, but also extremely calming and soothing.

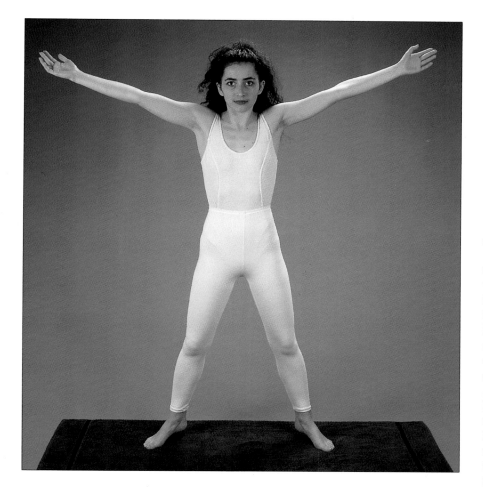

9 Move your legs further apart. As you breathe in, stretch out the arms, expand the chest, and rise up on to your toes (*left*); have the feeling of opening up the whole of the front of the body. As you breathe out, let your shoulders relax and drop, lower your heels on to the floor and pound strongly all over the upper chest (*bottom left*). This activates Ki in the whole body, and is good for waking up the system in the morning. It also helps move local energy blockages, trapped emotion or congestion in the chest. If you wish, you can add internal vibration by voicing a loud 'Aaaah' sound on each out-breath. Repeat the whole exercise three times in all.

10 Rub the cheeks vigorously (*below*) with alternating palm action. This particularly stimulates the lungs and breathing. It makes a good completion to the above sequence, or can act as a lead-in into the facial sequence on the following pages.

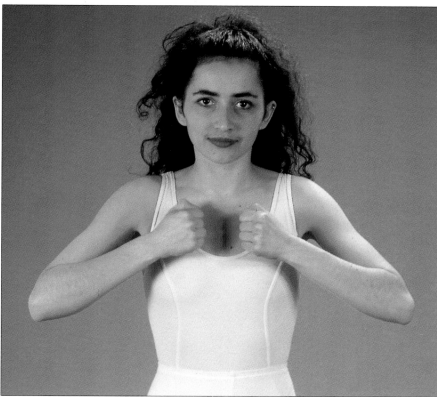

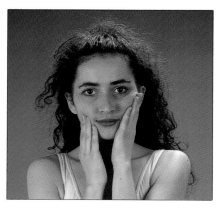

FACIAL SELF-SHIATSU

Many pressure points corresponding to different organs in the body occur in the face, so its treatment brings benefit to the whole system. It also releases facial tension, tones the skin and muscles, and brings extra circulation to the area. A daily facial treatment will help offset the effects of stress or ageing, and make you look consistently brighter and fresher.

The sequence here is an adaptation of lesson 10 in Part One, adding techniques around the eyes that are unsuitable to use on others; you may wish to refer back to the points marked on pages 93–96, and the notes on benefits associated with them. As usual, pressure is generally exerted on the out-breath, and everything is repeated three or more times.

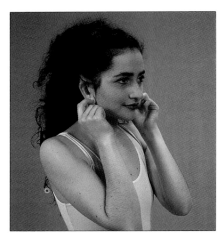

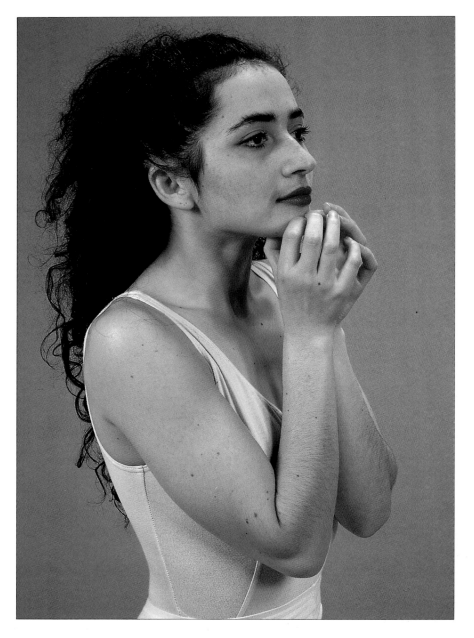

1 You can sit, stand or kneel to carry out this sequence. Begin by massaging the ears (*above*). Squeeze and pull them strongly, all around the outer ear including the lobes.

2 With your thumbs, press in under the chin (*right*). Move the thumbs simultaneously away from each other towards the ears, pressing under the edge of the jaw until you reach ears.

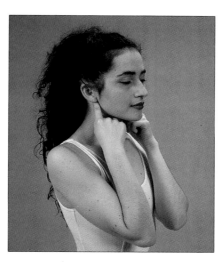

3 With the tips of your forefingers, press into the hollows that appear at the end of the jaw-bone when you open your mouth (*right*), just under the main part of the ear and behind the earlobe. Treating this point helps with metabolism and the distribution of heat in the body.

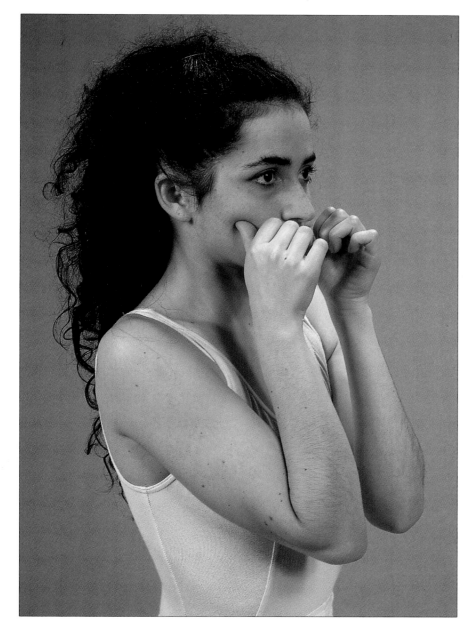

4 Starting just in front of the lower ear, press with your thumbs along the underside of the cheek-bone (*left*). Follow the lower edge of the bone until it disappears near the nose. Treating these pressure points is helpful for sinus and nasal congestion, facial tension and toothache.

5 With the tips of your forefingers, press into the two small hollows just to either side of the nostrils (*below*). These are the classical Shiatsu points for treatment of sinusitis; they also help with facial tension.

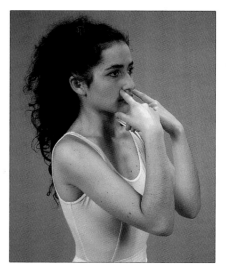

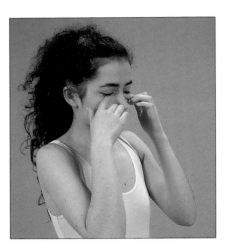

6 With the tips of your forefingers, press in under the eyeballs, between them and the sockets (*right*), working along from the inner to the outer corners of the lower eyelids. You may be surprised at how painless this exercise is, and how soothing for swollen or painful eyes it is; but do make sure that your fingernails are cut short and do not dig into the delicate skin here.

7 With the tips of the thumbs, press in over the tops of the eyeballs, between them and the sockets (*right*), working from the inner to the outer corners of the upper eyelids. You can also do pressure-point work at the two small hollows on underside of the brow, each about one-third of the way along from the inner end.

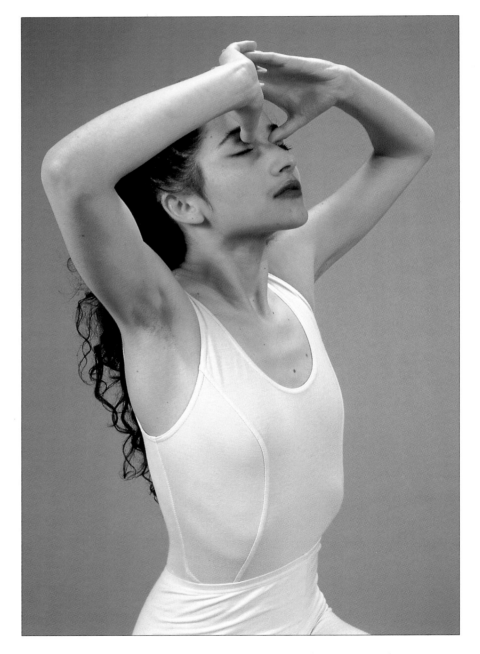

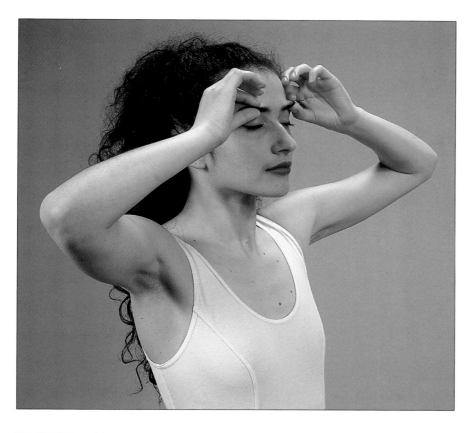

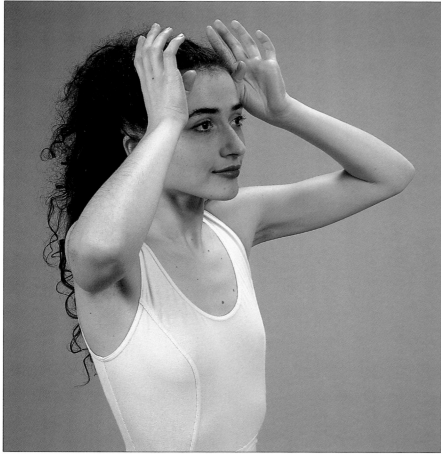

8 Pinch the eyebrows strongly between finger and thumb (*left*), moving from the inner to the outer corners. This adds to relaxation of the upper face.

9 Massage the forehead (*left*), by pressing in and drawing the base of the thumbs out over the forehead, towards the temples, lightly at first and then more strongly. You can finish with a similar but lighter massage here with the fingers laid flat and swept out in the same pattern.

10 Finally, massage the temples with the tips of the middle fingers. This completes the facial sequence.

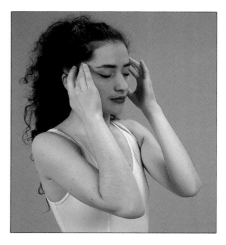

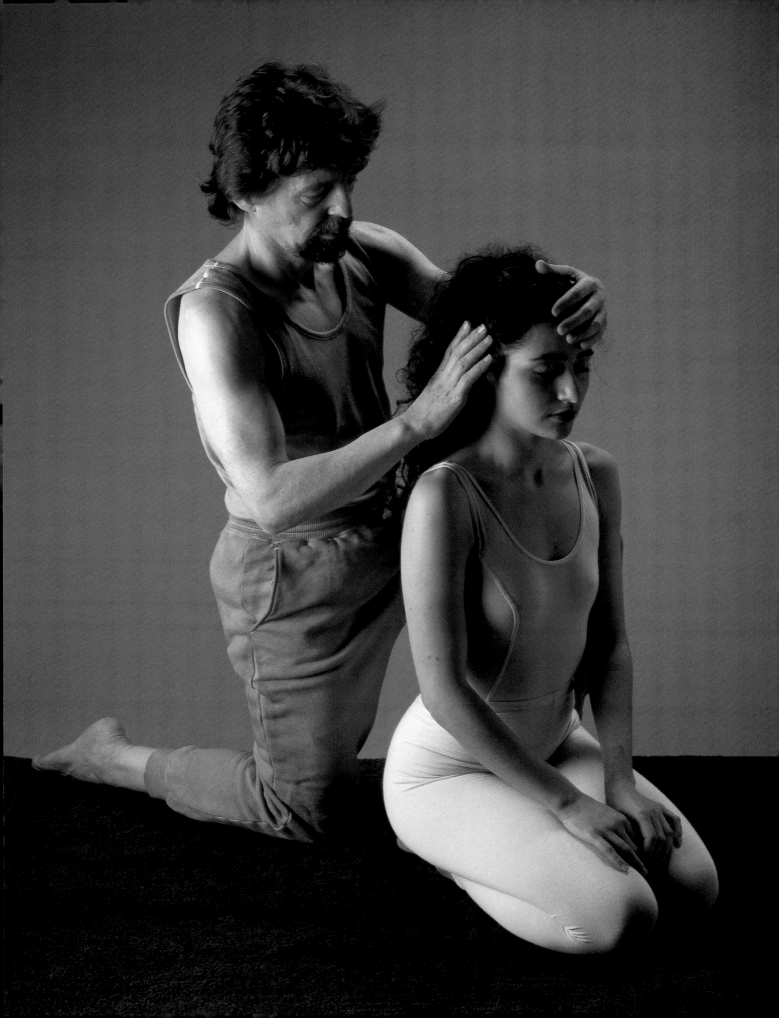

PART THREE

DEVELOPING YOUR TECHNIQUE

When you have practised the treatment sequence in Part One a number of times, you will find that you can follow it using only the illustrations. Once you are very familiar with the whole sequence, and are effectively incorporating the guiding principles of Shiatsu into your way of working, without thinking too much about them, you should find that the people you give Shiatsu to are receiving definite benefit from it. If so, then you are ready to develop your technique further.

There are four basic ways in which you can take your technique to a more advanced level: by developing your own internal energy awareness with breathing and visualization exercises; by improving your sensitivity to Ki flow in the body of the recipient; through studying the way Ki operates in the body, such as learning the paths of the channels, and the Chinese Five Element system; and by adapting the techniques that you have learnt to different individuals, and to treat specific health conditions.

These are all dealt with in this order in the following pages. You will probably find it best to take the material a little at a time, becoming familiar with it and weaving newly-developed skills into regular practice, rather than trying to take it all in at once. Once you are familiar with the more advanced techniques you may wish to pursue a more specialized branch of Shiatsu technique; this is best done by attending classes. Guidance on finding and choosing classes is given at the end of the section.

Left. *More advanced work*
can include adaptation or modification
of the basic treatment to suit individual
requirements or circumstances.

SELF-DEVELOPMENT EXERCISES

You will already have some experience of contacting your own Ki from your practice of Shiatsu so far. During the treatments you have given, hopefully you will have had some experience of the flow of Ki in your own body, and how that connects with the energy in your partner's body. The following exercises and guidelines are intended to help you develop that awareness. Breathing and visualization exercises are included, plus a simple exercise to experience your own energy in your hands.

Hara and breathing

As described in the Introduction, one of the most helpful habits to cultivate when doing a treatment is to focus attention and breathing in the lower abdomen, or hara. The hara contains the Tan Den, one of the seven major energy centres or chakras in the body, which have been used for thousands of years throughout the world in healing and spiritual practices.

You can think of the Tan Den as being located a couple of inches below the navel, in the middle of the body, a little forward of the spine. It forms the body's centre of gravity; focusing attention in this spot is widely used throughout the Orient in all kinds of activity where Ki is employed, such as in all martial arts, as well as in archery, the tea ceremony and even in flower arranging! Cultivating the ability to work with your attention here will greatly enhance your own calmness, concentration and 'centredness'. It will also help you to provide just what your partner's energy field needs, unthinkingly and instinctively, even if you are not able to detect this intentionally just yet. You will be consciously using your own Ki, and not just your physical strength and weight. If you develop this ability as second nature, it will also help bring these positive qualities to other activities in your life besides Shiatsu, including all kinds of physical activity or any interactions with other people, with powerful and far-reaching results.

This cultivation of hara focus can be done as a very simple exercise in its own right, as well as during Shiatsu practice. Just sit in a comfortable upright posture – the kneeling position (*below*), known as seiza, is ideal, but you can use any of the other sitting positions, which are shown at the beginning of lesson 1. Placing a cushion on top of your feet in the kneeling position can make sitting up straight more comfortable.

Allow all the different parts of your body to become completely relaxed. Focus attention in the hara, and feel yourself breathing into the Tan Den, deeply but in an unforced manner, and with a natural rhythm. Feel the abdomen swelling as you breathe in, and flattening as you breathe out. Placing your hands on your belly just below the navel will help this awareness. If you notice your attention wandering from the breath, just bring it gently back to this practice. If you are not used to abdominal breathing, continue for a couple of minutes.

To develop this exercise, you can try to feel the air, and Ki with it, flowing down into the hara as you breathe in. Hold the breath and concentrate on the energy there for a few seconds. Then let the breath out slowly, with your attention still on the Ki held in the hara.

As you breathe in again, sense that more energy is being drawn down, and continue in this way with a sense of energy building up and gathering in the Tan Den, for a few more minutes.

The whole exercise can be done for about five minutes daily, preferably

Left. *This position, known as seiza, is perfect for breathing into the hara.*

122

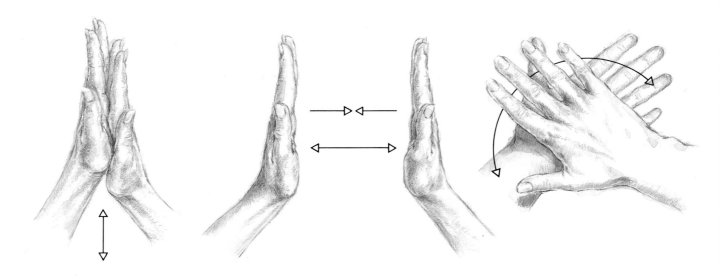

Above. *Rubbing the hands together stimulates Ki flow through them. You can feel the enhanced Ki as you move the hands together and apart* (top centre), *or pass one across the other* (top right).

when you are not too tired. It is also particularly useful in preparing yourself for giving a treatment, helping you to let go in your mind of everything else. Soon you will find that you can also cultivate hara awareness while doing all kinds of other activities, especially during simple, rhythmic actions such as walking, but you can even make use of it at such mundane moments as waiting in a queue.

It should be added that the Tan Den is just one of the chakras or energy centres found in the body that can be used as a focus in this way; some practitioners use the heart centre in a similar way. This is located in the middle of the upper chest area, again centrally between front and back of the body. The qualities and areas of life affected by this chakra include the emotions, compassion and relationships to other people. After getting used to working with and focusing in the hara you may wish to practise drawing energy into the heart centre in the same way, especially to cultivate working with altruistic intent or emotional healing. As an exercise for yourself, breathing into this area will also help you contact your own emotions, and can help heal difficult or painful relationships.

Alternatively, there is the brow chakra, or Third Eye, which is located behind the midpoint of the eyebrows. Focusing here, either as an exercise in itself or during treatment, will help develop potential for insight, intuition and psychic awareness.

Energy in the hands

This simple exercise is helpful in developing awareness of your own Ki and increasing the effectiveness of your treatments. It can be used before giving Shiatsu or self-treatment.

Sit or stand with the spine straight, and the body relaxed. Pay particular attention to the shoulders; if they feel tense, follow the corresponding self-treatment sequence on page 110. Then rub the hands together, with the fingers pointing upwards at the level of your face, and the whole of each hand making contact with the other, right down to the wrist. Do this for about 20 or 30 seconds, then separate the hands and hold them parallel to each other, about six inches apart. Do you feel any kind of sensation in them? Rubbing the hands together in this way stimulates Ki, which is often experienced as a sense of tingling, like an electrical charge, or sometimes like magnetic attraction or repulsion, or even like an almost solid ball of energy between the hands. Experiment by varying the distance between the hands, or moving them so that one passes the other, still with that space between, and observe the sensations. Closing the eyes can help. You may not feel these sensations at first, but if you practise the exercise you soon will. Even if the sensations are not apparent at first the Ki is still there, so it will still enhance your subsequent treatment.

A variation on rubbing the hands together, which some people find more effective, is simply to shake them vigorously for about half a minute, still with the shoulders relaxed, and with the wrists floppy. Then try moving the hands relative to one another (*see page 123*).

DEVELOPING SENSITIVITY TO KI

The techniques used in the basic sequence in Part One included overall stretches and some other instances where both hands or arms are used equally, but the predominant method that you have been using for palm and thumb work has been what is commonly known as 'two-hand work'. This title is somewhat misleading as it actually means that you are using the two hands simultaneously but in quite different ways; one is more passive and inactive and stays more or less in one spot, as the other hand moves along a line of points. This is particularly useful for rebalancing the energy between the two points of contact, and will help you develop sensitivity to what is going on in particular places.

If you keep practising your Shiatsu technique you will begin to notice that you encounter different 'qualities' of energy or Ki in the points where you apply pressure in the course of treatment. At the most obvious level, as discussed in the back sequence (*see page 34*), the body tissue overlying the area you are working on can have very different qualities to the touch – common impressions include tightness, openness, hardness or sometimes a kind of empty lifelessness. These are expressions of the Ki situation in that part of the body, relative to other parts. There is always some degree of relative imbalance or unevenness in the distribution of Ki, however slight – the body tissue will feel different from one area to another; and that is why we do Shiatsu – there will inevitably be some areas that lack Ki and others that hold excess. When you

become experienced in the technique of leaning into an area or point with your palm or thumb, you will soon be able to go below the surface of the person and contact the underlying energy, from which you can obtain a more specific sense of what is happening there in terms of Ki.

Tsubos

Points in Shiatsu are known as *Tsubos*, a Japanese word meaning 'vase'. This is because the impression on pressing on a Tsubo is, first of all, some resistance, which yields as the point is held, whereupon there is a feeling of 'opening out' under the thumb, before connecting with the 'bottom' of the point. This is illustrated in the diagram below; even if you do not experience these perceptions immediately, you will do so if you practise enough, and learn to locate points more precisely. What you are doing, in effect, when pressing and holding a Tsubo in this way, is connecting with the Ki underneath the point's surface, many Tsubos being 'gateways' into a Ki channel or meridian. The way you experience Ki in specific points is known as the Tsubo effect.

One of the main differences between acupressure or acupuncture and Shiatsu, and one of the great benefits of Shiatsu, is that you can actually treat any point on the body, and not just the ones that are on the classical channels. However, the classical points are more obvious to locate, more straightforward to treat, and easier to learn the effects of; so you will probably do best to focus on these at first. Later, you will find that you can apply the

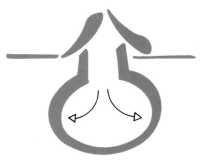

Above. *The Japanese written character for Tsubo shows how a pressure point is like a vase with a narrow neck and a lid on top.*

same principles in an almost infinite number of locations.

Kyo and Jitsu

When you locate a point, or Tsubo, and press into it, contacting the energy that lies under the surface, you will be aware of its particular quality. The terms Kyo and Jitsu are used to describe or classify the two extremes of qualities. Kyo is the quality of emptiness, indicating depletion, underactivity or lack of local energy, and Jitsu describes a sense of fullness, excess, overactivity or oversufficiency of Ki. They are relative rather than absolute values, used for comparison; and the conditions they describe are also dynamic, and always in a state of some degree of fluctuation, though some conditions can be very long-term. Distinguishing between whether energy is Kyo or Jitsu is very helpful, for it will help you to determine, first of all, what the existing situation is (diagnosis) and then what steps to take to remedy it (treatment). Pain or other evidence of disorder is often directly linked to the spot where imbalanced energy is detected in terms of Kyo or Jitsu, and can be directly treated there.

Kyo and Jitsu, as expressions of relative energy 'content', do not apply only between individual points, but also between different channels and the organ systems that go with them, as well as between different parts or zones of the body, and even between one whole person and another. Thus, in a particular person, the kidney meridian may be found to be the most Kyo; the lower body might be more Jitsu than the upper body; and the whole person could be judged to be relatively Kyo compared to most people – all these factors will influence the form of treatment you choose. Examples of the recognition and approach to such situations are given later, when we look at individual treatment.

Increasing your sensitivity to other people's Ki

Breathing into your hara and bringing Ki flow into the hands (see pages 122–3) also increase awareness of the aura or energy field that externally surrounds the body. You may wish to develop this awareness further to sense the aura around another person. After rubbing and/or shaking the hands, move one hand around the head, shoulder and upper body of your partner, who can be sitting. Make sure that you are relaxed. Again experiment with distance, and close the eyes if this helps. At a certain distance you may notice the sensation of entering the energy 'field'. Try this with different people – the strength and quality of aura varies hugely from person to person, and even over time. You may find that one of your own hands is naturally rather more sensitive than the other. With practice, you may find that certain parts of the aura are more intense or weaker than others, indicating areas of the body that may be holding an excess, or deficiency, of energy, which you can then take into account during your treatment.

KI IN THE HUMAN BODY

Oriental culture has developed a number of ancient classical systems of analysis for examining how energy works in the universe as a whole, and in the human being in particular. These are extremely helpful in preparing more advanced strategies for diagnosis and treatment. They include the Chinese model of the organ systems, the classical system of meridians and points, the laws of Yin and Yang and the Five Elements.

The vital organs

Classical Chinese medicine takes a somewhat different view of the body organs and their functions, from modern Western medicine. The traditional oriental view of the body is focused not only on each physical organ and its mechanical function, but on the different energy qualities of each system, and how these energies all complement each other and interact as a whole. Each of these organ systems includes a meridian, or channel along which its Ki flows in a particular direction; and from the point of view of both diagnosis and

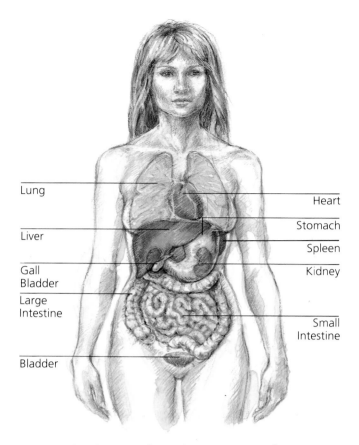

Lung

Liver

Gall
Bladder

Large
Intestine

Bladder

Heart

Stomach

Spleen

Kidney

Small
Intestine

Above. *This diagram shows the positioning of organs that have corresponding meridians. Note that the kidneys lie at the back of the rib-cage behind the other organs.*

healing these are more important than the organ themselves.

Relationships between the organs are also viewed differently in the classical Chinese system of medicine. The primary breakdown is not into functional groups such as stomach/ small intestine/large intestine, but into pairs of organs which are complementary and have a balance of energetic functioning between them; the pairs themselves are in turn ordered into a sequence through which there is an overall Ki flow. This is explained below. The positions of the major organs in the body are shown in the diagram above.

The energy channels

Awareness and understanding of the channels or meridians are vital to the development of your Shiatsu technique. They are usually considered to provide the most valuable guideline for where to apply treatment, and the effect it will have. The concept of meridians brings together the Classical Chinese system of vital organs and the oriental concept of Ki.

The meridians can be thought of as a web or network of energy channels, running through the body, connecting each organ system with the extremities of the body – the head, hands and feet. In classical oriental medical texts, they are described rather poetically as 'the web that has no weaver'. Where a channel runs near the skin surface, it permits treatment that will primarily affect the corresponding organ system.

There are fourteen major classical meridians in total. Ten of them are associated with the major physical organs and are paired, in keeping with the associations of organs through their complementary 'energetic' functions:

Lung with Large Intestine
Stomach with Spleen
Heart with Small Intestine
Bladder with Kidney
Liver with Gall Bladder

In addition to these, there are two more pairs of energy meridians which do not have corresponding organs in the physical sense, but are important nevertheless. These are:

Heart Governor and Triple Heater
Governing Vessel and Conception Vessel

The functions of all these organ systems are summarized below, and can be studied in more detail in the following pages. All the meridians, except the Governing Vessel and the Conception Vessel, have double channels that appear symmetrically on both the right and left of the body; when you treat them, you work on the channels on both sides. The Governing Vessel and the Conception Vessel have a single channel each, one running centrally down the front of the body, and the other running centrally down the back (*see pages 128 and 130*).

In fact, you have been working on almost all of the meridians already in the step-by-step sequence in Part One, and parts of them have appeared in the photographic superimpositions that showed you where to apply pressure. They have not been discussed in depth until now in order to encourage you to get an intuitive feeling for where to press, and to work with Ki in a tactile way, rather than being 'in the head' and using the mind too much.

Having practised the basic sequence, your Shiatsu technique will now be enhanced by having more detailed information about where to apply pressure, and about what the effects will be at the different points. Knowledge of the meridians also allows you to do specific treatment – for instance, if you know someone has weak intestines you can focus on that meridian – but it also makes it possible to get specific information about particular organs from what you detect from the state of the Ki in particular channels.

There is a definite direction of Ki flow in each of the meridians. Generally speaking, the flow is down the back of the body (as it appears when the arms are raised over the head) and the outside of the limbs, and up the front of the body and the inside of limbs. This dictates the pattern of treatment in Part One and self-treatment in Part Two. The exception is the stomach meridian, which runs downwards on the fronts of the legs. The routes of the meridians are shown schematically on the following pages. Some of the more important specific treatment points are also shown; how to locate them more precisely follows shortly. There is also an overall flow of Ki in the whole system, through one meridian after another, as shown in the list below.

The functions of the organ systems
The following analysis of organ systems gives an indication of its role in oriental terms. Each organ system and its related meridian has a common abbreviation, which is given in brackets after the full name below.

Lungs (LG): take in air and the Ki that it contains, converting them into Ki for body use and circulating it to the other channels; this meridian also supports mental positivity.

Large Intestine (LI): refers chiefly to the colon; it removes the fluids from food and excretes unwanted solid matter; also involved in issues of 'holding in' and of self-confidence.

Stomach (ST): prepares food for digestion and extracts Ki and nutrients, to be directed to the spleen or small intestine; is also related to functioning of the intellect.

Spleen (SP): transforms energy from food into Ki for the body, clears old cells from blood and plays a major part in the immune system. In Chinese medicine, it is grouped with the pancreas, which produces hormones and enzymes to aid digestion, and control blood sugar and fat metabolism; also governs the ability to mentally concentrate and analyze.

Heart (HT): circulates blood and controls blood vessels. The heart is seen as the seat of the consciousness and feelings.

Small Intestine (SI): receives food from the stomach, separates and absorbs nourishment, before passing the remainder to the large intestine and bladder; also influences mental discrimination.

Bladder (BL): temporarily stores and excretes waste fluids; also associated with courage.

Kidneys (KD): store and provide Ki for the organs and for the fundamental life processes of birth, growth and reproduction; they also maintain fluid levels and eliminate toxic waste products. The kidneys also affect will-power.

Heart Governor (HG): Supports the heart functions, including blood circulation; influences human relationships. (Also known as Heart Protector or Pericardium.)

Triple Heater (TH): distributes Ki through the body and regulates heat; enables emotional interaction with others. (Also known as Triple Burner or Triple Warmer.)

Gall Bladder (GB): stores bile which the liver produces, and supports the liver functions; is also involved in making decisions, going forward and taking action.

Liver (LV): stores blood, and facilitates all flow of Ki in the body; removes toxic substances from the small intestine; also associated with creativity, humour and planning.

Governing Vessel (GV): controls the meridians of the front of the body and inside of limbs.

Conception Vessel (CV): controls the meridians of the back of the body and outside of limbs.

Each organ system further affects particular emotional states as well as other aspects of physical health. These are discussed more fully under The Five Elements on pages 131–2.

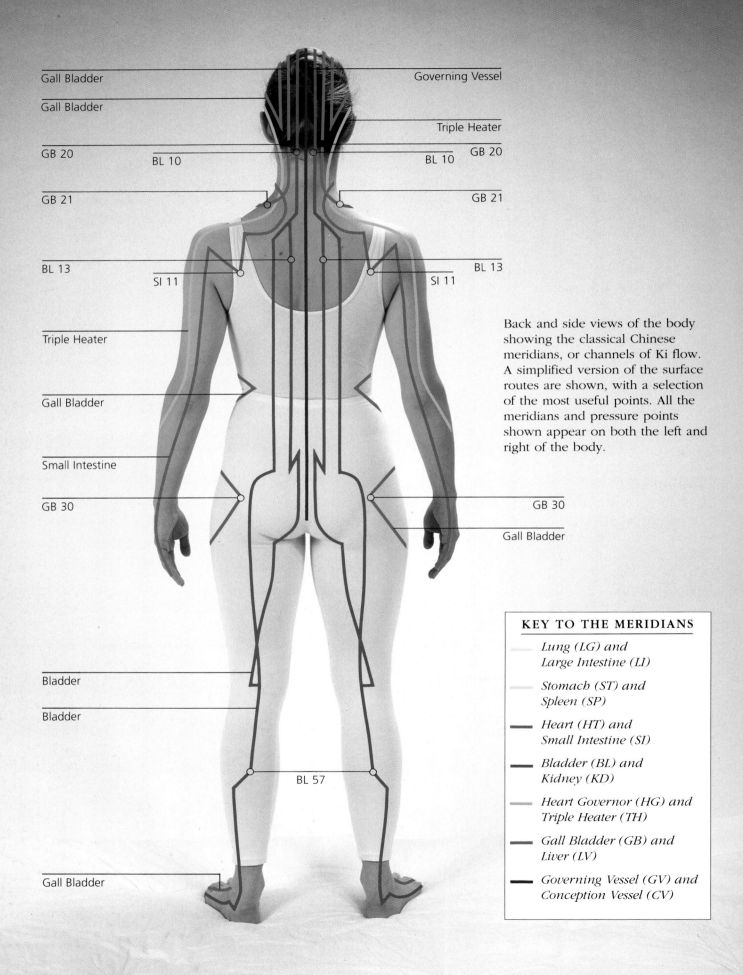

Gall Bladder

Gall Bladder

GB 20　　　　　BL 10

GB 21

BL 13　　　SI 11

Triple Heater

Gall Bladder

Small Intestine

GB 30

Bladder

Bladder

Gall Bladder

Governing Vessel

Triple Heater

BL 10　　GB 20

GB 21

BL 13　　SI 11

GB 30

Gall Bladder

BL 57

Back and side views of the body
showing the classical Chinese
meridians, or channels of Ki flow.
A simplified version of the surface
routes are shown, with a selection
of the most useful points. All the
meridians and pressure points
shown appear on both the left and
right of the body.

KEY TO THE MERIDIANS

*Lung (LG) and
Large Intestine (LI)*

*Stomach (ST) and
Spleen (SP)*

*Heart (HT) and
Small Intestine (SI)*

*Bladder (BL) and
Kidney (KD)*

*Heart Governor (HG) and
Triple Heater (TH)*

*Gall Bladder (GB) and
Liver (LV)*

*Governing Vessel (GV) and
Conception Vessel (CV)*

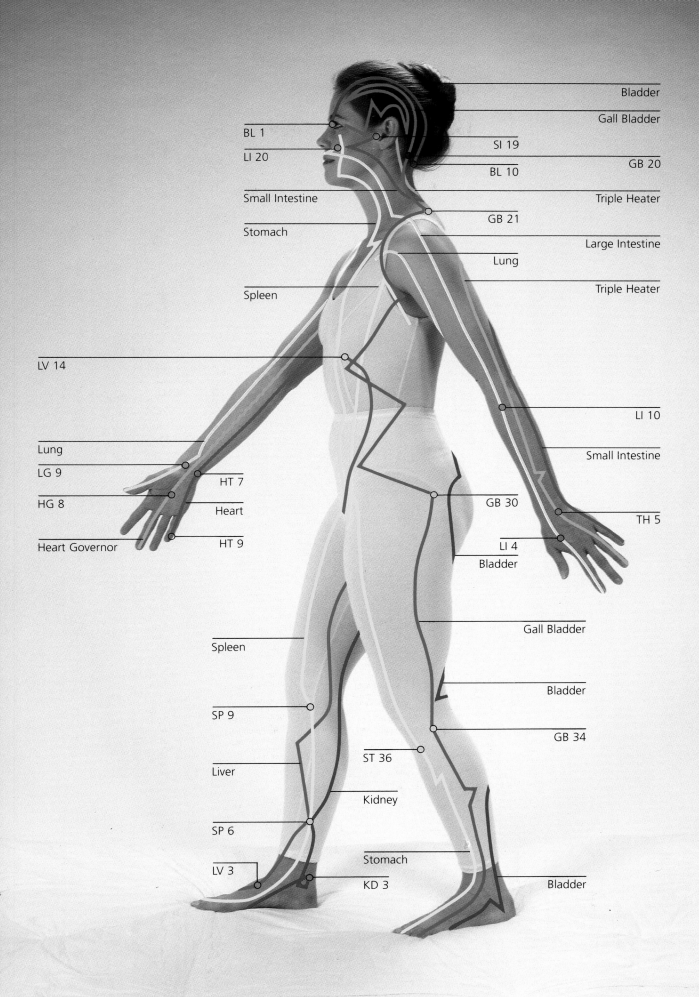

Bladder

Gall Bladder

BL 1

LI 20

SI 19

GB 20

BL 10

Small Intestine

Triple Heater

Stomach

GB 21

Large Intestine

Lung

Spleen

Triple Heater

LV 14

LI 10

Lung

LG 9

HT 7

Small Intestine

HG 8

Heart

Heart Governor

HT 9

GB 30

LI 4

Bladder

TH 5

Gall Bladder

Spleen

Bladder

SP 9

GB 34

Liver

ST 36

Kidney

SP 6

Stomach

LV 3

KD 3

Bladder

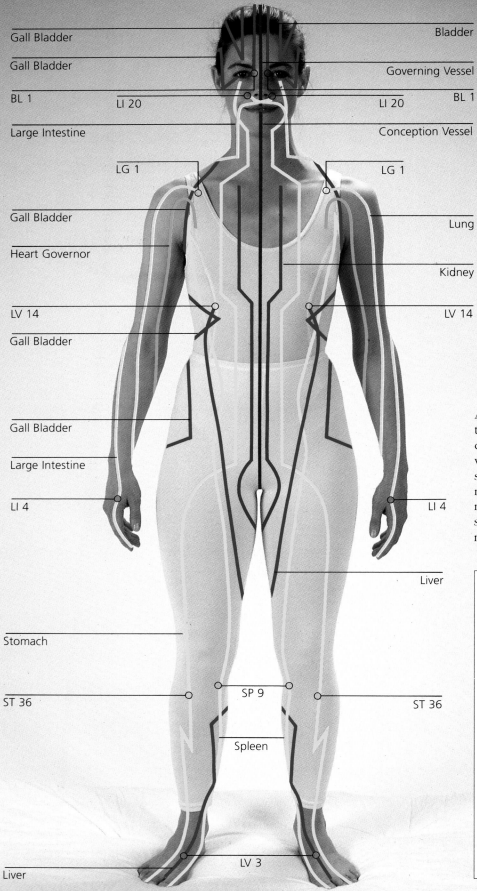

Gall Bladder
Gall Bladder
BL 1
LI 20
Large Intestine
LG 1
Gall Bladder
Heart Governor
LV 14
Gall Bladder
Gall Bladder
Large Intestine
LI 4
Stomach
ST 36
SP 9
Spleen
Liver
LV 3

Bladder
Governing Vessel
BL 1
LI 20
Conception Vessel
LG 1
Lung
Kidney
LV 14
LI 4
Liver
ST 36

A front view of the body showing
the classical Chinese meridians, or
channels of Ki flow. A simplified
version of the surface routes are
shown, with a selection of the
most useful points. All the
meridians and pressure points
shown appear on both the left and
right of the body.

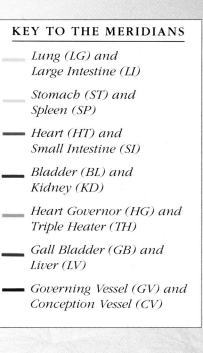

KEY TO THE MERIDIANS

*Lung (LG) and
Large Intestine (LI)*

*Stomach (ST) and
Spleen (SP)*

*Heart (HT) and
Small Intestine (SI)*

*Bladder (BL) and
Kidney (KD)*

*Heart Governor (HG) and
Triple Heater (TH)*

*Gall Bladder (GB) and
Liver (LV)*

*Governing Vessel (GV) and
Conception Vessel (CV)*

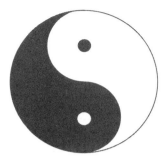

Left. *The well-known symbol for Yin/Yang shows how each force tends to contain an element of its opposite.*

Yin and Yang

The concept of *Yin* and *Yang* is another distinctively oriental way of understanding how energy works, and one that is fundamental to the whole of Eastern cosmology, and to the oriental understanding of how the body organizes itself.

The concept of Yin and Yang was first set down thousands of years ago in the ancient Chinese classic, the *I Ching*, or Book of Changes, but awareness of it probably goes back further still. All energies and phenomena in the universe can be classified as predominantly either more Yin or more Yang. But each phenomenon contains an element of both, as expressed in the famous symbol (*above*), and it is important to remember that the analysis can only be used comparatively. No single phenomenon or force is absolutely Yin or Yang, but only by comparison with or in the context of another phenomenon or force. Furthermore, the manifestation of the two types of energy is dynamic and always changing and interplaying, as in ongoing natural cycles such as day and night, winter and summer, birth and death and so on. Thus the qualities of Yin and Yang respectively are usually described in terms of corresponding pairs of opposite adjectives – light and dark, hot and cold, male and female and so on. Yang energy is more dynamic, active and outwardly manifest; Yin energy is more passive, internalized and inherently less evident. Yin and Yang are 'complementary opposites', and they always tend to operate together to bring any situation into a state of balance or resolution. Thus an extreme Yin phenomenon will become less extreme by attracting an element of Yang energy, and vice versa.

Examples of complementary opposites

More Yin	More Yang
Stillness	Movement
Shade	Sun
Cold	Warmth
Darkness	Light
Passive	Active
Inward	Outward
Invisible	Visible
Soft	Hard
Wet	Dry
Female	Male

In Shiatsu terms, the concept of Yin and Yang is helpful in a number of ways. Firstly, as all Ki arises as a manifestation of the interaction of Yin and Yang qualities, learning to distinguish between these relative qualities as they appear in the body can deepen our understanding of the way Ki operates there. The meridians themselves are divided between Yin and Yang: the Yang channels run down the back of the body and outer edges of the limbs, and are associated with the more 'solid' or yang organs, such as spleen, heart and kidneys; Yin channels are located on the softer front of the body, and serve the more Yin, more 'hollow' organs like stomach, small intestine and bladder. Thus we can better understand the organ and meridian pairings. The meridians are divided between Yin and Yang as follows:

More Yin	More Yang
Large Intestine	Lung
Stomach	Spleen
Small Intestine	Heart
Bladder	Kidney
Triple Heater	Heart Governor
Gall Bladder	Liver

Secondly, we can use Yin/Yang understanding to apply the appropriate form of treatment or correction, for instance by reducing extremes of Yin or Yang. We will look at this further when we consider principles of individual treatment. Yin/Yang is also a fascinating concept in itself, and if you study it further there is no end to the ways you can find to apply it to other departments of your life. Finally, the concept of Yin/Yang leads us into the classical Chinese Five Element system.

The Five Elements

This is yet another component of oriental cosmology that provides a distinctive way of looking, in more detail, at just how energy works. And yet again, it can be used to understand the whole of creation, but here we will be concerned with applications of particular relevance to Shiatsu.

The cycles of nature have already been cited as an illustration of the interaction of Yin and Yang energies, and the Five Element system uses them as a descriptive device too. In fact, a more accurate title would be The Five Phases of Energy Transformation; the so-called 'elements' are really only symbols of these phases.

The ongoing cycle of energy from Yin to Yang and back to Yin again in the cycle of the natural year, for instance, can be drawn as a circle, and then further sub-divided into five distinct phases that interact with each other and in relation to the whole. The phase known as Water represents the stillness – like winter – before the rising, expanding energy of the springtime, which is represented by Wood. The energy of the earth's atmosphere reaches the climax of this rising tendency in the summer phase, which is termed Fire, at which

point the expanding tendency is replaced by the late summer quality of settling or descending. This is the Earth stage. The further condensing and contracting tendency of autumn is the Metal phase, which leads again into winter and Water.

Any number of other models can be drawn on to illustrate the possibilities of applying this analysis, but the natural cycle of plant growth will serve here to give a little more idea of the unique energy qualities of each stage. The dormancy of plants, with all the energy passively stored in the roots while snow covers the ground, is the classic image for Water. Outwardly, it looks as if nothing is happening, but subtle preparation is taking place for the next phase, Wood. The energy of Wood is the unstoppable, bursting, upward and outward growth force of plants coming up from the ground, or budding on branches. This in turn develops into the full growth and flowering peak, which is the Fire phase; at this point, the growth energy is more fitful and beginning to falter, like individual flames that lick upwards energetically, but each die down immediately. Earth energy, next, is when energy is gathering inwards to the swelling of fruit; this has, by nature, a more stable quality. The Metal phase is the setting of seed, the most contracted manifestation of plant energy, which then lies dormant in turn as Water time comes round once more. This sequence is shown in the diagram left.

This elegant schema can also be applied to the organization of energies in the body – for instance to the system of Ki and the energies of the organs – which thus provides another sophisticated tool for enhancing diagnosis and treatment. Each element or energy phase controls a particular pair or pairs of organs. Water energy governs the kidneys and bladder; Wood characterizes the liver and gall bladder; Fire energy is the dominant nature of the heart and small intestine, as well as of the heart governor and triple heater. The stomach and spleen are governed by Earth energy, and the lungs and large intestine by Metal. We can then use an understanding of each element to further our understanding of the organs,

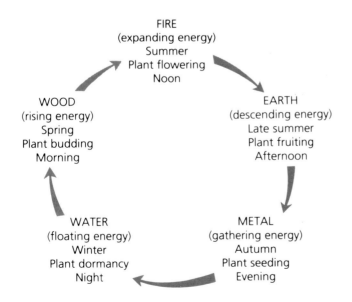

Above. *The classical Chinese system of Five Elements for analysis of the five phases of the transformation of energy, their respective associated qualities, and phenomena in the human body and the natural world.*

Below. The inter-relationship between the Five Elements and their associated emotional states – the Control Cycle, shown by inner, straight arrows, and the Support Cycle, shown by the outer, circular arrows.

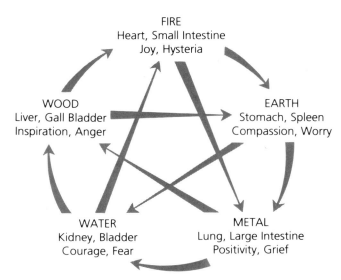

FIRE
Heart, Small Intestine
Joy, Hysteria

WOOD
Liver, Gall Bladder
Inspiration, Anger

EARTH
Stomach, Spleen
Compassion, Worry

WATER
Kidney, Bladder
Courage, Fear

METAL
Lung, Large Intestine
Positivity, Grief

including how they relate to different seasons, for instance. Furthermore, we can identify different emotional states that are associated with each energy phase, and with each set of corresponding organs.

Finally, we can gain an understanding of how the organ systems dynamically interact with each other from the inter-relationships of the elements. This interaction is in two distinct patterns. Each element has a relationship first of all with those two others which are adjacent to it on the progressive cycle, and secondly with those two which are opposite, across the circle. The relationship with adjacent elements concerns their complementary nature, and is known as the Support Cycle; thus, in the symbolism of nature, wood burns to create fire, fire produces ashes that nourish the earth, earth contains the ores of metals, metal melts into the liquid state of water, and water nourishes the growth of wood. The relationship between opposite elements, by contrast, concerns their antagonistic or restraining potential, and is called the Control Cycle; so water dampens fire, fire melts metal, metal cuts wood, wood penetrates earth, and earth channels water. If the energy of an element is weak, it can be enhanced or increased by input from its supporting element, but if it is oversufficient it can be limited by input of energy from the controlling element.

All of these interactions are shown in the second Five Elements illustration (*left*). The goal of Shiatsu treatment is to enable the recipient to harmonize with the energy of the environment and of life. The Five Element analysis is extremely useful in this; how to apply it will be discussed in more detail under Individual Treatments, below.

TREATING THE INDIVIDUAL

There are three broad ways in which Shiatsu benefits the body's internal energy patterns:
1 removing local blockages to the natural flow of Ki;
2 improving the overall level or quantity of Ki if it is deficient or excessive;
3 restoring the relative balance of Ki between specific places.
Detailed awareness of these patterns only comes with experience and practice, but a regular whole body session using the techniques and quality of treatment set out in Part One will go a long way towards making these improvements. This is because the body has an ability to restore its own internal balances between any two points or zones, simply with the help of basic palming techniques, for instance. However, as you become proficient you will want to tailor your work to the needs of the recipient; some guidelines follow to help you make individual distinctions in your work, and these will also provide a basis for further study and knowledge.

Every person is absolutely unique in their state of being; furthermore, everyone finds themselves in a different state from year to year, day to day and even moment to moment, whether it is slightly or distinctly. So no two Shiatsu treatments need ever be identical, although there has to be a standard format to follow when learning. On top of this, there are many aspects to our condition of health or well-being – not only physical but also of an emotional, psychological and even spiritual nature. Shiatsu, like any other truly holistic therapy, can be helpful in treating all these aspects. In this instance we will mainly go into the treatment of physical and emotional issues, but general purpose Shiatsu will naturally also benefit the majority of people's sense of mental well-being, inner peace and ability to adjust to life's challenges. Where there are very serious disorders, whether mental, emotional or physical, you are strongly advised against giving treatment yourself; instead you should refer the person to a fully qualified Shiatsu practitioner. Contact numbers for organizations worldwide, who can help you find a practitioner, are given on page 142.

There are two stages to adapting your Shiatsu to suit an individual – firstly diagnosis, or working out what the person is experiencing; and secondly, treatment, or addressing what you have discovered. In practice these processes intertwine continuously throughout a session, for as you give Shiatsu you will inevitably be getting information back; but some particular methods of diagnosis can be studied in isolation. At first these techniques will require conscious mental activity on your part, but when you are thoroughly familiar with them they will become second nature, increasingly instinctive and intuitive, thus allowing you to be centred more in the hara, and less in the head.

Actually, diagnosis need not be the clinical activity that it sounds. As human beings, we are naturally interested in how other people are – as most of our conventional forms of greeting show. And we are naturally skilled, too, at judging this for ourselves. We notice when people do not look well, and we are intuitively aware that what we see on the outside reflects what is going on inside, even if it is only that someone is looking a bit pale or washed-out. Oriental diagnosis is really an amplification of this principle, with particular aspects developed into highly sophisticated arts. So, there is facial diagnosis, voice diagnosis, diagnosis by posture, by pulse or even by the condition of the fingernails, to name but a few methods. This is in addition to what we can gather from more conventional observation of outer symptoms, and from what our prospective client can pass on to us from other health practitioners. Last but not least, we will learn by touch and energy sensing, as we actually get on with the treatment – for instance, the sense of Kyo or Jitsu (see page 125). No-one uses all methods of diagnosis at once; rather, it is usual to make a preliminary assessment using a preferred technique, then verify this with one or two other methods, and decide on treatment accordingly. Noticing an energy imbalance in this way, and treating it before outward symptoms have had a chance to manifest, is clearly an advantage that methods such as Shiatsu offer.

In keeping with the oriental way of doing things, the first thing to look at is the overall picture before going into the detail – and gear the overall quality of the treatment to this. The large, tense, extremely muscular person may not even feel the type of pressure or stretches that could be too much for the light frame of a more delicate or frail person. Looking a little deeper, we can say that a person with an overall more Jitsu condition – energetic, active and with more evident Yang qualities in the body, mind and emotion – will benefit from a more sedating type of treatment. This involves working with pressure that is quick and strong, thus drawing out, releasing and dispersing the excessive Ki quality. Stretching, shaking and squeezing are also helpful local sedation methods, which may sometimes include working against the direction of Ki flow in the meridian. A person who is overall more Kyo, on the other hand – who seems comparatively weak and lacking in vitality – will require more tonifying: working in a slower, gentler way but with longer holding, especially in the direction of flow of the meridians, to support and amplify existing Ki. Applying the principles of Yin and Yang to specific symptoms, we can say broadly that a more Yang condition or illness is characterized by symptoms that are more acute and active and more easily perceived, and is often accompanied by tension, stress or fever; whereas predominantly Yin symptoms are more often hidden in the body or otherwise difficult to detect specifically.

The same principle can be applied at other levels, for instance in different body zones within one person. The upper or lower body, or some parts of the spine, may be comparatively Kyo (seeming weak, lacking in muscle tension, unnaturally soft, cold or with a lifeless quality) or Jitsu (excessive muscle tension, feeling hard, hot) and can be treated accordingly with tonifying or sedation. Jitsu areas by their very nature tend to stand out, attract attention and generally be more obvious.

Individual meridian or Tsubo quality can be distinguished and treated likewise; local pain is a good indicator that there is a Kyo or Jitsu imbalance in that area. When treating meridians that are paired, with one channel in each leg for example, both branches should be treated. One approach often used by professionals is to find the most Kyo and most Jitsu channels and focus particularly on treating them, or even simply focus on tonifying the most Kyo, so that Jitsu naturally balances itself in the process. Sedation of the points can be enhanced if necessary by circular movements of the thumb on the point, and excessively empty points can be toned by holding for ten or fifteen seconds, or even up to several minutes in extreme cases. Strong stretches are inappropriate for an extreme Kyo condition. *(For treatment of specific ailments see pages 139–41).*

Working with pressure points

In Part One, you have already treated a considerable number of specific points in the course of following lines of treatment suggested by the photographs with superimposed pressure points. In the following pages more information is provided on locating points, or Tsubos, much more precisely, and learning more and more about the individual ability of particular Tsubos to help you develop your technique further.

Naturally, these points will present you with a wide range of possible sensations, depending on a number of variables – including what is going on at the skin surface, what is happening with overlying muscle tone, whether the underlying condition is more Kyo or more Jitsu, and so on. Some helpful pointers

concerning these phenomena follow. Shiatsu teachers, however, have become aware that everyone has an innate sensitivity for picking up on underlying energies, although it is usually fairly unconscious until it is developed by deliberate study. Students who are absolute beginners can somehow intuitively find points and even instinctively go to the points that most need treatment; so try not to suppress that inbuilt, tactile capability as you learn techniques with your intellectual faculties. As you practice more, you will often find that when checking how points feel along a certain meridian, for instance, the hand just stops at a particular point which is somehow 'different'. This is the instinctive energy-sensitive faculty at work, and it can definitely be hindered by an overly-active mind. It is enhanced, on the other hand, by the techniques mentioned at the beginning of this section, notably relaxation in your own body and focus in the hara.

When you are working with points, communication with your partner can help you a lot. Pressing and holding on Tsubos gives the receiver a particular sensation, which regular Shiatsu recipients will soon come to recognize – that particular kind of 'tenderness', already mentioned, which even when it is somewhat uncomfortable is not quite the same as other pain. So your partner can often let you know when you are exactly on a Tsubo, and also give you feedback on the amount of pressure you should use, and what the effects are of pressing deeper or holding longer.

Useful pressure points

A selection of well-known and useful points on the meridian system are set out on pages 136–9, and these will enhance your technique and also help you treat a range of common complaints. Effective treatment can be given almost anywhere on the body, but over the millennia during which Chinese medicine has developed, particular points have been found to be consistently beneficial in very distinct and particular ways. This selection is by no means exhaustive – classical acupuncture identifies at least 365 points, though not all are regularly used – but it will serve to introduce the subject of point location and treatment, and provide a substantial degree of treatment opportunity. When you have studied some or all of these, you will be able to go back to places in the Part One treatment sequence where they occur, and incorporate accurate and knowledgeable location into your work.

These points are identified sequentially by the meridian on which they lie. Treatment of a point not only affects the meridian and the corresponding organ, but also brings benefit to the local area, as well as to a number of other body functions; it can also relieve disorders seemingly quite unrelated (in Western medical terms) to the main associated organ system. For instance, SI 11, located on the shoulder-blade, is on the small intestine channel; it also helps with shoulder pain and lung problems. Explanation of the subtle and often complex relationships of oriental medicine are beyond the scope of this book, but will be found in standard texts on Chinese medicine or acupuncture theory (*see Further Reading, page 142*). Many of them also have traditional Chinese names, such as 'Bubbling Spring' or 'Palace of Weariness', which you may also like to study, as they can give a profound insight into the energetic qualities and effects.

The three meridian charts on pages 128-30 will give you an approximate idea of where the point is to be found, while the photographs of the local areas, together with the notes below, will enable more precise location. The unit of measurement most commonly used for point location, relative to prominent features of body geography such as joints or muscles, is the width of the thumb (known as one cun). Strictly speaking, this is the recipient's thumb width, so if you have tiny dainty hands and are treating a person with very large ones (or vice versa) you should take this into account. The width of the four fingers is also used for larger distances; this is equivalent to three cun.

The best way to find a point is to use this information for approximate location, and then move around the area with the thumb, pressing until you feel the point opening out under your thumb – the 'Tsubo effect' described on page 124. While you are still a beginner, it is wise to consult with your partner who will be able to help you locate the precise spot.

Do please remember to observe the cautions mentioned here for some of the points.

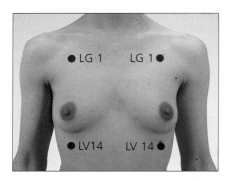

directly below the nipples, between the sixth and seventh ribs down from the collar-bone. You should be able to feel an indentation here.
For chest constriction, difficult breathing, coughing and rib pain, lactation problems, belching and nausea.

Lung Meridian – LG 9: on the crease on the inside of the wrists, in the indentation between the bones below the base of the thumb.
For shallow or painful breathing, coughing, pharyngitis, lethargy, wrist pain; first-aid point for reviving from unconsciousness.
Heart Meridian – HT 7: in the crease of the wrists, in the indentation below the corner of the palm on the little finger side.

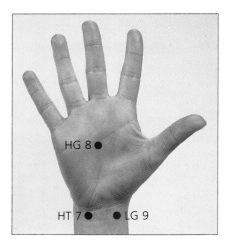

For insomnia, irritability and hysteria; first-aid point for reviving from unconsciousness.
Heart Governor Meridian – HG 8: in the middle of each of the palms.
For physical exhaustion – primary point for enhancing energy levels.

Lung Meridian – LG 1: on the upper chest, one thumb width below the projecting point of each collar-bone, in the hollow at the corner of the gap between the first and second ribs.
For common cold, cough, asthma, breathing difficulties, chest pain, chest congestion.
Liver Meridian – LV 14: just above the lower edges of the rib-cage,

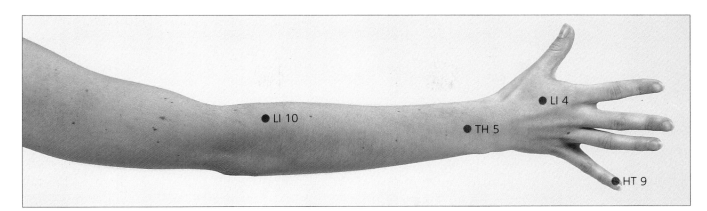

Large Intestine Meridian – LI 4: on the back of the hands, on the middle of the muscle in the web between the thumb and forefinger. *For improving the functioning of the intestines, coughs, sinusitis, controlling pain in upper body, especially the face (toothache, for example), and general well-being.* **Caution: Do not treat during pregnancy**

Large Intestine Meridian – LI 10: on the outer fore-arms, one and a half thumb widths down from the end of the crease (which appears in the crook of the elbow when the arm is bent). The point is approximately in line with the index finger. *For pain and fatigue in the arms, releasing muscular spasm, to relieve sore-throats and for general well-being.*

Heart Meridian – HT 9: on the insides of the little fingers, near the bottom corner of the nail. *For anxiety and hysteria; first-aid point for angina and heart attack.* **Triple Heater Meridian – TH 5:** on the back of the arms, two thumb widths above the wrist crease. *For tinnitus, ear infections, migraine headaches and feeling cold in the body.*

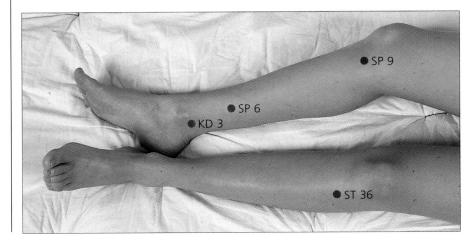

Large Intestine Meridian – LI 20: near the corners of the nose, in the small hollow just outside the nostrils' widest point. *For sinus and nasal congestion, and for facial pain.*

Bladder Meridian – BL 1: marginally above the inner corner of the eye; use the little finger to press inward and upward, as the thumb is too clumsy for this precise point. *For swollen or tired eyes, poor vision and insomnia.*

Stomach Meridian – ST 36: on the outside of the shin-bones, four fingers width below the kneecap, in the depression at the outer edge. *For tired legs, poor appetite, and to promote general well-being.*

Spleen Meridian – SP 6: inside of shin-bones, four fingers width above the knobble of the ankle-bone. Also a point on the kidney and liver channels, which intersect with the spleen channel here. *For menstrual and other female reproductive problems, digestive problems, overweight and insomnia.* **Caution: Do not treat during pregnancy**

Spleen Meridian – SP 9: inside of shin-bone, just below the knee. *For anxiety, hysteria and knee pains; first-aid point for angina and heart attack.*

Kidney Meridian – KD 3: on the inside of the ankle-bone, half-way between the Achilles tendon and the tip of the ankle-bone. *For kidney malfunctioning.*

137

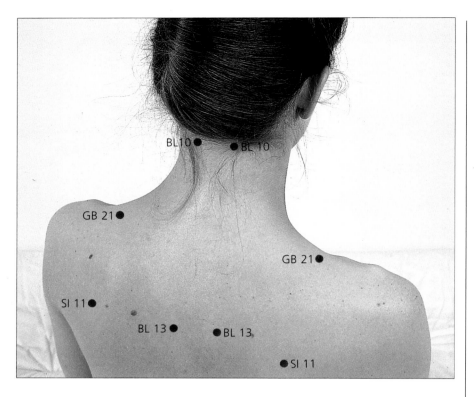

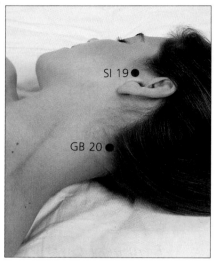

Small Intestine Meridian – SI 11: on the upper back, in a depression at the centre of the shoulder-blades. *For frozen shoulder, shoulder pain, neuralgia; also helpful for any lung problems, such as breathing difficulties, asthma or coughing.*

Bladder Meridian – BL 10: at the back of the head, just below the base of the skull, one thumb width out from the spine on either side. *For headache, neckache, insomnia and nasal blockage.*

Bladder Meridian – BL 13: one and a half thumb widths to each side of the spine, level with the space between the third and fourth thoracic vertebrae. *For lung problems, such as asthma, coughs, bronchitis, pneumonia and breathlessness; also any bladder problems, as well as lethargy and melancholia.*

Gall Bladder Meridian – GB 21: on the top of the shoulders, straight up from the nipples. *For frozen shoulder and shoulder pain, and to improve lactation.* ***Caution: Do not treat in case of pregnancy***

Small Intestine Meridian – SI 19: in the indentation that appears just in front of the middle line of the ears, when the jaw is slightly dropped. *For tinnitus and hearing difficulty.*

Gall Bladder Meridian – GB 20: just below the base of the skull, in the hollow that is found there, to the outside edge of each side of the trapezius muscle. *For common cold, headache, sore and swollen eyes and neck tension.*

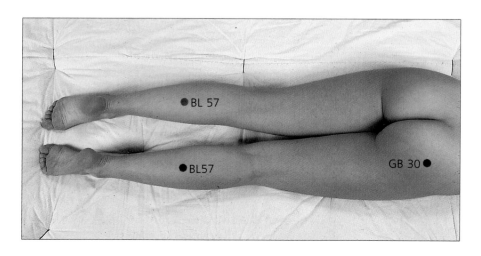

Bladder Meridian – BL 57: on the backs of the legs, in the centre of the calf muscle, half-way between the back of the knee and the heel. *For muscular tension, cramp, stiffness or tiredness in the lower legs, varicose veins, sciatica and haemorrhoids.*

Gall Bladder Meridian – GB 30: in the large indentation of the muscle on the side of each buttock, one-third of the way from the top of the femur to the coccyx. *For lower back pain, sciatica, arthritis or rheumatism in the hip.*

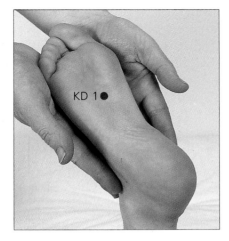 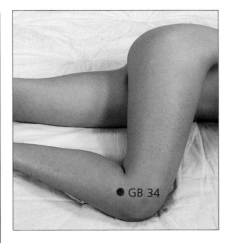 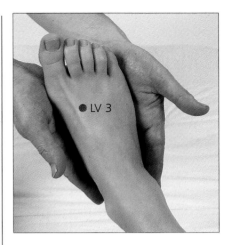

Kidney Meridian – KD 1: on the sole of the feet, half-way across the width and one third of the way from the top of the middle toe to the bottom of the heel.
For menstrual pain, dizziness and general vitality; also a first-aid point for unconsciousness.

Gall Bladder Meridian – GB 34: on the outside of the legs just below the knee, in the bony indentation below the kneecap. To treat this point, make sure that the leg is raised in the 'recovery' position.
For headaches, leg weakness, knee problems and ankle pains.

Liver Meridian – LV 3: on the top of each foot, one and a half thumb widths in from the web between the first and second toes towards the in-step.
For headaches, dizziness, muscle tension and cramps.

Treatment for specific ailments

If your partner is suffering from particular health problems, it is often possible to gear the treatment to these, or at least include some specific procedures. Some examples are given here, including self-help advice that can be given to the receiver. You will find that some points listed below form helpful elements of an overall approach to a particular problem, even though they are not a specific effect of that particular pressure point as mentioned above.

Common Cold and Flu: standard Shiatsu treatment with particular emphasis on the back, neck and head is generally helpful for a cold or flu, serving to shift blocked and stagnated Ki, to strengthen immunity and to move toxins into the bloodstream and thus out of the body. The treatment often pushes the cold on more quickly, and 'brings things to a head'. Particular treatment of the lungs is beneficial, and working in the Spleen channel on a regular basis can enhance more long-term immunity. Particular points that can be incorporated into the treatment include LG 1, LG 9, SI 11, BL 10, BL 13 and GB 20; and LI 4 and LI 10 to ease associated aches and pains. For coughs, use LI 4, BL 13,

LV 14, and nasal congestion LI 20, BL 10. See below for sinus congestion and headaches.

Sinusitis and Sinus Congestion: treatment of the lung and large intestine meridians is usually helpful, including extra attention to LI 4 and especially LI 20.

Asthma: treat the lung meridian, as well as the neck, shoulders, upper back and rib-cage points. LG 1, BL 13 and GB 21 are particularly beneficial. Since asthma is closely related to allergies, food and other intolerances (especially dairy food, for instance) may be checked to support self-help measures.

Constipation: naturally the main approach will be to physically treat the abdomen in the circular, clockwise direction shown on page 71, as well as the large intestine meridians in the arms, but treatment of the shoulders will help too. LI 4 is a particularly useful point, which can also be pointed out to the receiver for self-treatment, as it is easy to find. In fact it is valuable to show clients how to do abdominal self-massage and self-treatment (*see pages 103–19*), which is very straightforward and greatly promotes bowel regularity. Dietary and exercise recommendations may also be appropriate.

Diarrhoea: give light Shiatsu to the abdomen, as well as to the large and small intestine meridians, plus ST 36 and KD 1. The receiver should keep the hara warm, fast if he or she is not too weak, and take care to replace lost fluids.

Fatigue: give general Shiatsu and abdominal treatment; work on the spleen meridian if there is wide fluctuation of blood sugar (tiredness in the afternoon after eating, for example) and the kidney channel if there is evidence of deeper depletion of resources. HG 8 and ST 36 can be useful for short-term effects. BL 13, LI 10 and KD 1 can be used on a regular basis to promote longer-term vitality.

Headaches: contrary to the pharmaceutical companies' apparent beliefs, there are many different kinds of headaches, which have different causes and therefore require different approaches to treatment. They vary greatly in terms of location, duration and sensation. Generally speaking, however, there is nearly always an element of stress, with corresponding neck or shoulder muscle tension and obstruction of blood flow to parts of the head. The most important item on the agenda is to find out and remove the underlying cause, but treatment of the neck, shoulders, upper back and affected part of the head is usually very helpful, as indeed is full body treatment. Points that are effective in at least some cases are ST 36, GB 20, GB 21, BL 10, LI 4, and LV 3. Treatment of migraine is highly possible with Shiatsu, but is generally a more specialized subject than can be treated here, although TH 5 is helpful in some cases.

Insomnia: one of the commonest benefits that people report from Shiatsu is that they sleep better after a treatment, even if that was not the problem they came to solve. During treatment, receivers nearly always become extremely relaxed, including those who usually find this very difficult. Again, it is important to discover the underlying cause of poor sleep and

deal with it; but Shiatsu treatment can usually provide some improvement in sleeping patterns, whereupon the person will be in a better position to find out what is wrong and do something about it. Whole body Shiatsu is undoubtedly beneficial, but particular attention can be paid to the kidney and bladder meridians, as well as to treatment of the abdomen and feet, plus BL 10, HT 7, KD 1 and SP 6. Self-help suggestions might include appropriate exercise, avoidance of stimulants such as caffeine and not eating late in the evening.

Back Pain: the simplest initial approach can be to treat Tsubos in the area of the pain with a view to correcting excessive Kyo or Jitsu, avoiding pressure on the spine itself if it is painful; and to release associated tension that you may find in other zones in the back. Recurring problems in the back usually reflect underlying weakness in the local organs; lower back pain, for instance, often means problems with the kidneys or bladder. So checking and treating whichever organs require treatment will usually also help with a back problem. GB 30 is useful for lower back pain, and the point in the centre of the back of the knees is a traditional Tsubo for relieving all kinds of back pain. Never apply pressure directly to injured areas, such as slipped disks.

Menstrual Problems: abdominal Shiatsu can be helpful, but avoid strong pressure if it feels excessively uncomfortable. Treat the kidney, bladder and spleen meridians, and especially SP 6, which is a good point to show receivers for self-treatment, as well as KD 1.

Treating the emotions

One way of relating a treatment to the receiver's emotional state is to use the Five Elements system (*see pages 132–5*). Some simple applications of these principles are suggested here.

Broadly speaking, you can use knowledge of a person's predominant emotional condition to indicate the likely organ system that is most imbalanced, which can then be checked by other diagnostic criteria. This can be ascertained by observation or by questioning the client. These associations between organ systems and emotional patterns are set out in the diagram on page 133. So, if the predominant negative emotion at the time is anger or extreme impatience, then the first organ system to look at would be the liver and gall bladder (Wood). If the person is experiencing inexplicably deep melancholy, however, then the lung and large intestine (Metal) would be indicated. If there is such an emotional pattern that is very long-term and deep-seated, then we would suspect a correspondingly profound, perhaps even constitutional, imbalance in that organ system. If that diagnosis seems to be confirmed, for instance by touch diagnosis, then a treatment can be carried out with particular attention to treating those meridians and points.

However, the Five Elements system offers several other avenues of approach to treatment besides this most simple and direct one. These derive from the two ways that the Elements, or stages of transformation of energy, relate to each other, as already described – the Support Cycle and the Control Cycle. Wood energy, for instance, is supported by Water energy and in turn supports Fire energy; and it is inhibited by Metal and conversely inhibits Earth. These interactions afford subtle but powerful additional methods of aiding or affecting the Ki in the organ system in question.

If we take the case of liver disorder (Wood) for instance, and find that liver energy is more Kyo, we can work on that meridian with toning to strengthen it; but we can additionally work on the Water channels (kidney and bladder) in order to enlist the enhancing quality of the Control Cycle action. Even working on Metal energy can contribute in some degree. If, on the other hand, the Wood Ki is found to be more Jitsu, the most direct tactic is to sedate those channels, but another option would be to work on the element that limits Wood energy, namely Metal, via the lung and large intestine. Again, in the case of Wood Kyo, it may be found that Metal is excessive or Jitsu, in which case sedating the Metal will reduce the over-riding effect it is having on Wood. These more indirect methods can often be even more powerful than the more direct approach, because they are more holistic and tend to bring the entire system into balance. The use of the Five Elements can be a lifetime study in itself, and there is a whole school of thought in acupuncture that is based on it. References are provided on page 142 for those who wish to study it further.

How often to give treatment

For most people, the ideal frequency of treatment is about once a week, but if you have friends or family who wish to receive Shiatsu more often, it will benefit them more. In the professional context the same is recommended, although some clients may only be able to afford two-weekly visits. Once the client has obtained relief from his or her specific ailments, or recovered their general health, monthly or more occasional sessions can be recommended to maintain health.

Giving suggestions for health

When you have practised Shiatsu for some time, you will become aware – if you have not done so already – that the condition of health in which people find themselves is not something that comes out of the blue, but is mainly the result of the way they lead their lives. The exercise we take, the food we eat, our lifestyle and the kinds of influence we expose ourselves to, even down to the films we watch, all have a great bearing on the well-being of our body, mind and spirit. And insofar as we can choose these things, there is always something we can do that will improve our condition.

As you begin to address particular ailments, Shiatsu will enable you to treat the underlying Ki situation rather than the superficial symptoms. As your experience increases, you will gain more insight and begin to make yet more underlying connections with the causes operating in a given case. Many practitioners see it as part of their work to provide holistic recommendations relevant to the circumstances. Appropriate Shiatsu treatment that is accompanied by the recipient's own measures to improve their condition produces by far the most profound and dramatic progress.

RESOURCES

The following information provides some guidelines on the different types of Shiatsu practice available and how you should go about choosing a school or practitioner.

Different styles of Shiatsu
Shiatsu is not a uniform technique, but a rapidly evolving approach to bodywork characterized by different originating influences and developing strands. Students who wish to pursue Shiatsu further should look into the various approaches available today, and choose one that suits their purpose and temperament. Notes on some of the more common 'styles' follow.

Zen Shiatsu is the name given to the style developed by Shizuto Masanuga, who proposed the treatment of meridian 'extensions' beyond those recognized in the classical Chinese view. He also developed the widely-accepted 'two-hand' style, where one hand moves, applying pressure, while the other provides stationary support or 'listening', and the Kyo/Jitsu tonification and sedation principle.

Namikoshi Shiatsu was developed by Toru Namikoshi, who worked on integrating traditional Shiatsu with Western medicine from the 1920s onward. This style of Shiatsu is characterized by applying pressure to specific reflex points that relate to the nervous system, rather than to the classical Ki channels.

Macrobiotic Shiatsu makes use of the classical meridians, with additional input from Macrobiotics. Shizuko Yamomoto is one of the most influential teachers of this approach; her 'barefoot' style, as its name implies, is less analytical than some, bringing in considerable use of the feet.

TCM-based Shiatsu, or Traditional Chinese Medicine Shiatsu is taught in a number of schools, especially those whose teachers are also acupuncturists. This technique is based on the principles of Traditional Chinese Medicine.

Five Element Shiatsu is an approach to Shiatsu that emphasizes the Five Element system of diagnosis and treatment, particularly with respect to the emotions.

Hybrid Techniques are combinations of Shiatsu with other forms of therapy, notably healing with the hands, or traditional Japanese 'Palm Healing'.

Acupressure is akin to Shiatsu, but concentrates on treatment of the classical 'fixed' Tsubos; most Shiatsu styles incorporate this method, but focus at least as much on the whole channels, also incorporating a variety of other techniques or analyses.

Choosing a school or practitioner
If you are considering a school or teacher, you should always consult them about their basic approach, which will probably bear some resemblance to one of those mentioned above. You also need to check qualifications of teaching staff. Standards are set within many countries by recognized organizations (*right*), and are currently being harmonized within Europe and internationally. These organizations govern publicity, education and ethical standards for Shiatsu in their areas, and supply information on schools, teachers and practitioners.

In the UK the Shiatsu Society sets standards for teachers and practitioners. Students of Shiatsu must gain 500 hours of study with registered teachers over a minimum period of three years, before they can apply for assessment by the Society for entry to the professional register. Teachers must spend at least two years as registered practitioners before they can apply to join the teachers' register. Teachers must be registered for five years before they can become principal of a registered school.

Gerry Thompson teaches Shiatsu with The Wilbury School of Natural Therapy and The Devon School of Shiatsu. He also practises from his home in Brighton, England. His details are:
Gerry Thompson BSc Hons, MSc, MRSS
  Brighton Media Centre, 9 Jew Street,
  Brighton BN1 1UT
  Tel/Fax: (01273) 206000

Contact organizations
Information about Shiatsu practitioners, teachers or schools is available from the following associations; European contact addresses are available from The Shiatsu Society (UK). These details were correct at the time of going to press.

United Kingdom
The Shiatsu Society, 5 Foxcote, Wokingham, Berks RG11 3PG
Tel: (01734) 730836

United States
American Oriental Bodywork Therapy Association, 50 Maple Place, Manhasset, New York, NY 11030
Tel: (516) 365 5025

American Shiatsu Society, 44 Pearl Street, Cambridge, MA 02139

Canada
Shiatsu Association of Ontario, PO Box 695 Station P, Toronto, Ontario, M55-244
Tel: (416) 762 2260

Australia
Shiatsu Centre of South Australia, 98 Waterfall Gully Road, Burnside, SA 5066
Tel: (08) 338 1267

Shiatsu Therapy Association of Australia P.O. Box 1, Balaclava, Vic. 3183
Tel: (03) 525 8474

Further reading
Goodman, Saul. *The Book of Shiatsu*, New York, Avery, 1991

Jarmey, Chris and Mojay, Gabriel. *Shiatsu, The Complete Guide*, London, Thorsons, 1991

Kaptchuk, Ted. *Chinese Medicine: The Web that has no Weaver*, London, Rider, 1983

Lundberg, Paul. *The Book of Shiatsu*, London, Gaia, 1992

Masunaga, Shizuto and Ohasi, Wataru. *Zen Shiatsu*, Tokyo, Japan Publications, 1977

Matsumoto, K. and Birch, S. *Five Elements and Ten Stems*, Boston, Paradigm Publications, 1983

Namikokoshi, Toru. *Complete Book of Shiatsu Therapy*, Tokyo, Japan Publications, 1981

Ohashi, Wataru. *Do-it-yourself Shiatsu*, London, Allen & Unwin, 1977

Tara, William. *Macrobiotics and Human Behaviour*, Tokyo, Japan Publications, 1984

Yamomoto, Shizuko. *Barefoot Shiatsu*, Tokyo, Japan Publications, 1979

INDEX

ACKNOWLEDGEMENTS

I wish to thank warmly all the many people who have contributed directly or indirectly to the production of this book. These are some of them:

Those who have taught me Shiatsu over the past fifteen years, in particular Shizuko Yamomoto and Saul Goodman; other members of the Shiatsu community who have given advice or support, especially Elaine Liechti, Oliver Cowmeadow and Paul Lundberg; as well as other teachers who have opened up the mysteries of healing in general and the Orient in particular to me – Herman and Cornelia Aihara, Michio Kushi, Bill Tara and Louise Haye, to name but a few. I am also appreciative of students who have enrolled on courses, and their enthusiasm over the discovery of Shiatsu. My clients, too, have contributed by enabling me to pursue this deeply satisfying profession.

Due to the high design and illustration content, this book has been a team effort more than most books are. I am particularly grateful to all the publishing personnel, whom I now number among my friends, that have made the experience an exciting, creative, co-operative, sociable and almost exclusively joyful one! I thank Zoë Hughes and Hilary Krag for their day-to-day work on editing and design respecively; Elaine Partington for her overall design vision; and Ian Jackson, for deciding that a Shiatsu book of this kind was a good idea, and that I might be the man for the job. It was a fine experience, too, working with the photographer, Sue Atkinson. The models, Chloë, Matthew, Alex and Dervaragh were enthusiastic even during the long-held poses. The whole thing has been a lot of fun.

Finally I would mention my Mum, who put up with me 'not getting a proper job', and my Dad who was himself a natural healer; and Elaine Bellamy who has supported me emotionally and gastronomically throughout this project.

EDDISON · SADD EDITIONS
Art Director Elaine Partington
Art Editor Hilary Krag
Photographer Sue Atkinson
Illustrator Sharon Smith
Graphic linework Anthony Duke
Editor Zoë Hughes
Proofreader Barbara Nash
Indexer Dorothy Frame
Production Hazel Kirkman and Charles James

Futon Supplied by the Futon Company,
169 Tottenham Court Road, London W1P 9LH
Tel: (071) 636 9984